Revitalize Your Life

The Anti-Inflammatory Cookbook for Beginners with 1500 days of Recipes to Heal and nourish every cell of your body + 21 day meal plan

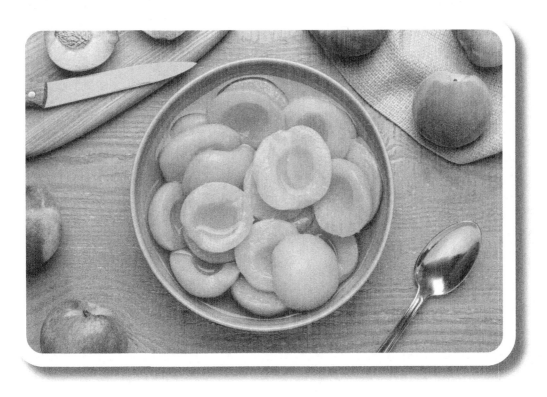

Becca Russell

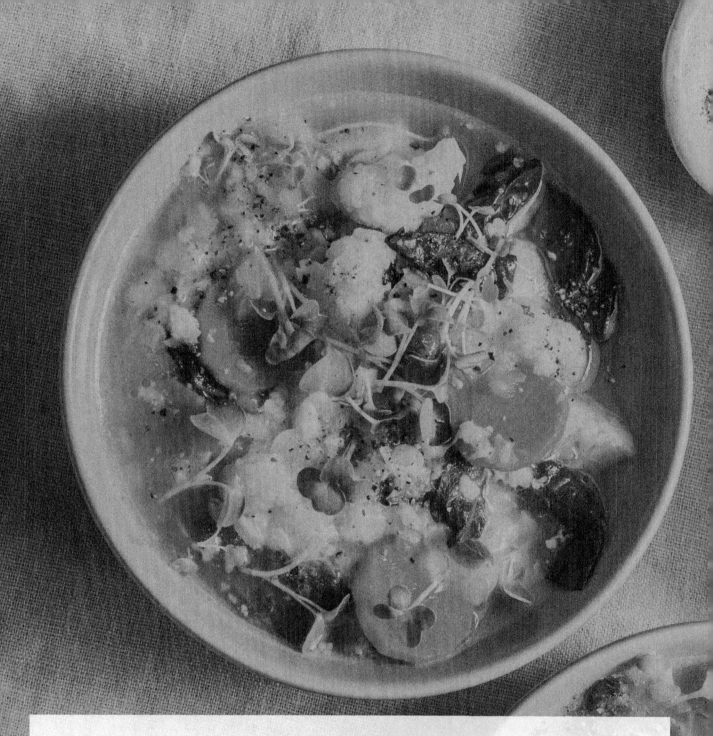

TABLE OF CONTENTS

TABLE OF CONTENTS

TABLE OF CONTENTS

TABLE OF CONTENTS

TABLE OF CONTENTS

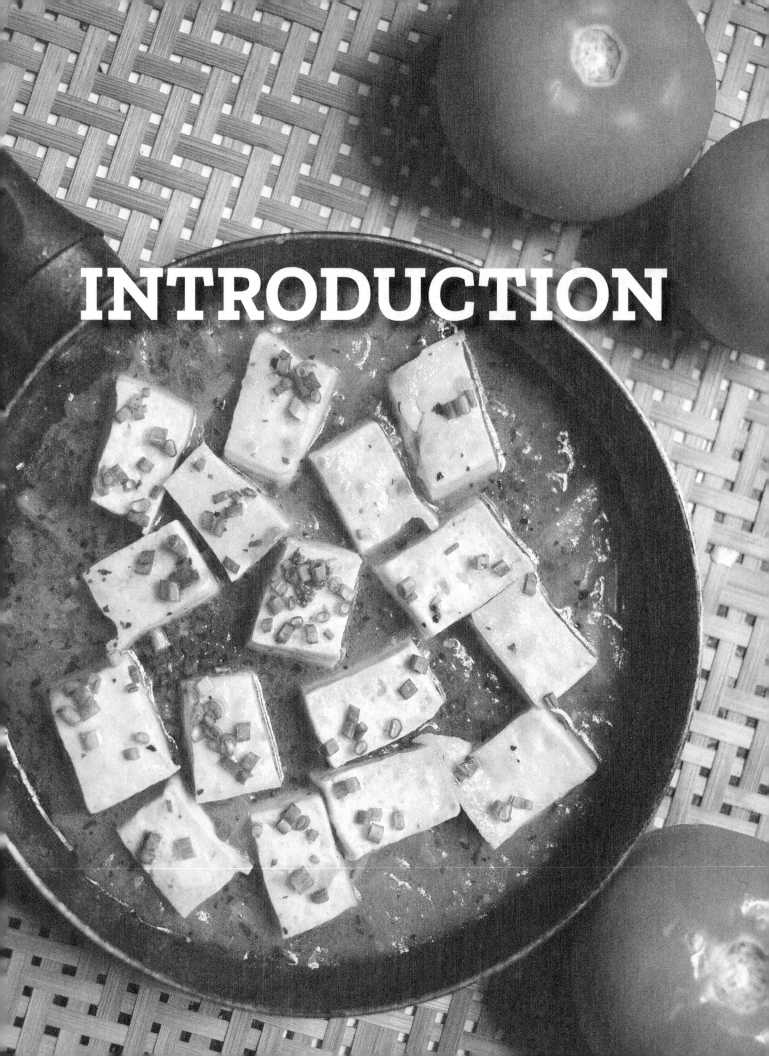

INTRODUCTION

"The silent killer"

That's what many scientists call it.

In the world, 3 out of 5 people die from a disease linked to this factor.

That's over 96,000 deaths every day.

Thirty-four million a year.

But the truly shocking fact is another.

This killer is "silent" but actually is plain to see if you know what to look for.

We all have it before our eyes and often we even live with it, without realizing.

What is it?

Chronic inflammation.

Recent research has correlated this problem with diseases as diverse as:

- Cancer
- Hepatic steatosis
- Kidney disease
- Hypertension
- Heart attacks
- Allergies
- Diabetes
- Asthma
- Rheumatoid arthritis
- Dementia.

Some scientists call chronic inflammation "the central mechanism" of Alzheimer's since this condition appears to be related to the chronic inflammation of nerve fibers.

However, I have some good news for you today.

It's in fact possible to both prevent and reverse the inflammatory process.

And as several studies show, one of the most effective strategies to do this is through the right diet.

So, today I want to disclose to you the two mechanisms of the anti-inflammatory diet – as well as the foods to avoid, and those to favor.

But above all, in this recipe book you will find tons of yummy recipes that will help you prevent or reverse chronic inflammation in just 3 months.

All without sacrificing taste and the pleasure of eating.

First, however, let me share the causes of the inflammatory process – and what you can do right now to counteract the problem.

1. What is chronic inflammation?

In this section, I want to show you what inflammation is, how it develops, and what symptoms to watch out for to recognize and stop it in time.

I will also reveal the difference between the two main types of inflammatory processes:

- Acute;
- Chronic.

But first of all, what is inflammation?

It's a natural process of the body, meant as a defense mechanism.

In case of injury or infection, it singles out and eliminates the harmful agent.

At the same time, it removes damaged tissues and promotes healing.

Therefore, inflammation is a beneficial process for our body and a crucial one for our survival.

Still, when the situation gets out of hand, this mechanism can damage our own bodies.

To better explain this concept, we divide the inflammatory process into two types.

- Acute inflammation: it has a maximum duration of a few days. It is the defense process by which our body removes harmful agents and repairs tissues. This inflammation is called "high grade". It manifests itself with recognizable symptoms such as sore throat, itching, redness of the eyes, or swelling. The situation resolves in a very short time.
- Chronic inflammation. Chronic inflammatory diseases are related to many millions of the world's deaths. They can go on for years without you even noticing. This is because their symptoms are often disguised as unimportant issues, so many people do not recognize them.
- It is therefore a subtle process that wears out your body from the inside, continuously and inexorably. Doctors also call this "low-grade inflammation".

Now that I've shown you the difference between the two types of inflammatory processes, I'm going to tell you how chronic inflammation is triggered, what its symptoms are, and the risks it exposes you to.

Let me try to explain its workings in the simplest way possible.

So, let's start with the basics.

When an inflammatory response starts in your body, all its related processes are triggered:

- Vasodilation, which means widening of your blood vessels,
- Increased tissue permeability, which could be described as more 'leakage' from your body tissues and organs,
- and White blood cell production. White

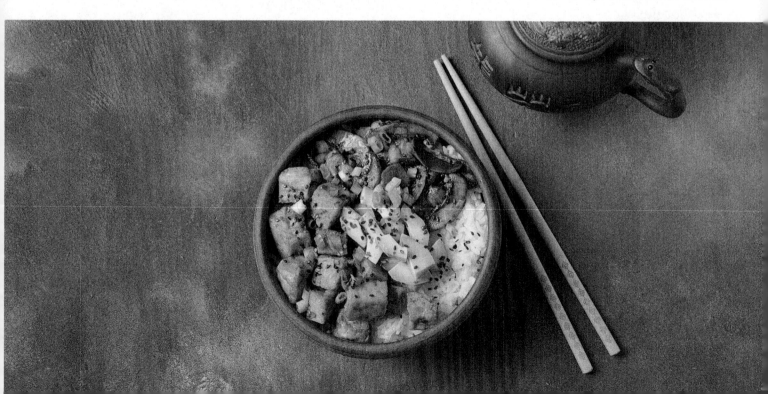

blood cells are what your body produces to fight infection, the "good soldiers" whose task is neutralizing pathogens.

Some of these "good soldiers" are called macrophages.

Their purpose is phagocytize the enemy cells – which is a particular kind of biological process to eliminate unwanted cells.

At some point – due to one of the causes that I will discuss in the next chapter – this inflammatory process gets out of hand.

The mechanism morphs from "high grade" inflammation to "low grade" inflammation.

Therefore, the initial symptoms fade, but a feeling of latent discomfort remains.

There is one particular aspect to emphasize.

Cytokine production increases at this stage.

What is it?

It's like messengers, whose task is to communicate with other cells to initiate the immune response.

At this point, your body increases the production of macrophages – the aforementioned "soldiers" with the task of tackling or phagocytizing pathogens.

The problem arises right here.

Once the cause of the inflammatory process has been eliminated, your body starts attacking healthy cells instead.

In turn, this mechanism increases inflammation and the body then sends more "soldiers" to try to defeat the enemy.

This creates a self-feeding vicious circle and inflammation becomes chronic.

So, if you – or one of your loved ones – develop symptoms such as:

- Tiredness
- Fatigue
- Loss of weight
- Weight gain
- Allergy
- Water retention
- Headache
- Sleep Disorders

… Then be alert.

Indeed, these are some of the subtle "red flags" of chronic inflammation.

In the next two sections, I will reveal the 3 mechanisms behind this process – and the habits to prevent or reverse the inflammatory process.

2. The 3 Mechanisms of Chronic Inflammation

In this chapter, I will quickly and easily reveal the main causes of chronic inflammation.

The following are all things you may already know, but maybe you still don't know how they can cause such a serious problem.

1. Stress

I'm sure you've heard of stress before.

But you may not know that this condition is linked to the development of about 90% of all diseases, as shown by a 2017 study published in the National Library of Medicine.

In our ancestors, stress occurred in fight-or-flight situations.

During an event such as a clash, the body triggers a series of reactions:

- Increased blood pressure;
- Increased blood sugar (the level of sugar in the blood);
- Release of cortisol and adrenaline (both inflammatory hormones);
- And many more.

All these reactions are meant to make the body more alert and responsive.

When unrelated to some actual danger, but only due to a state of anxiety that lingers throughout the day, if unmitigated this process leads to inflammation.

In ancient times, the emergency situation was resolved in a short time and the inflammatory process was therefore acute.

Today, however, we are no longer stressed about a fight, but because of everyday events: the mortgage to pay, work, differences of opinion with a partner, and so on.

Therefore, our body is in a permanent state of stress and constantly releases hormones such as cortisol and adrenaline, creating a state of chronic inflammation.

Or in other cases it keeps our blood pressure and blood sugar high, leading to diabetes and heart problems.

Just think, the risk of a heart attack is two and a half times higher in people with chronic inflammation.

2. Metabolic syndrome

The second factor is metabolic syndrome, linked to diet and a very important hormone: leptin.

When we are full, leptin sends a signal to a receptor in the brain and alerts it to activate a sense of satiety.

That's how we know we have had enough to eat and finish the meal.

However, unlike in ancient times, today we no longer eat for survival alone.

Nowadays we eat for pleasure, or because

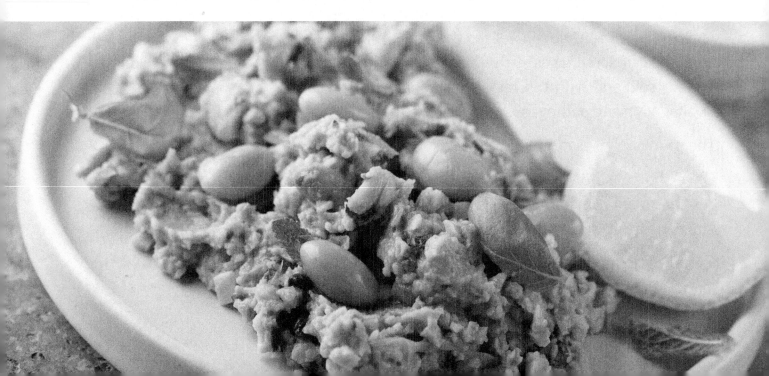

we are depressed, or stressed.

And what happens in such scenarios?

Our leptin levels rise dramatically until they peak.

At this point, the receptor in the brain is silenced.

I mean, it's like it no longer notices that you're full, and so it doesn't trigger a sense of satiety.

As a consequence, excess food and calories are transformed into fat.

This is where the problem arises because fat releases cytokines, or messengers of the immune response.

All this increases chronic inflammation, in a vicious circle.

But that's not all.

In fact, as shown in a 2019 study published in the National Library of Medicine, bad eating habits are linked to the development of 35% of cancers.

3. Lack of physical activity

This aspect is linked to the previous one.

In fact, it is clear that on average, sedentary people have a higher percentage of body fat.

And as I explained before, fat tissue is one of the causes of inflammation.

But that's not all.

Physical inactivity is extremely dangerous because it increases the risk of diseases re-lated to the chronic inflammatory process.

What am I talking about?

Cardiovascular diseases, for example, are 90% more likely to affect a sedentary person than an active one.

Again, 40% of patients with cognitive problems have chronic inflammation.

And physical inactivity plays a key role in this situation because it prevents the body from producing certain anti-inflammatory substances.

But more about that later.

Now, however, you need to know a very important fact.

These three causes have one crucial aspect in common: the production of free radicals.

In a nutshell, they are molecules that damage your body.

Now, however, I want to reveal the 5 habits to help you reduce the production of free radicals – and therefore prevent (or reverse) chronic inflammation.

3. The 5 habits to prevent or reverse inflammation

Now, I'm going to show you the habits to prevent chronic inflammation or cause it to regress.

But that's not all.

In fact, they will improve your overall health, reducing the risk of diseases such as cancer, diabetes, hypertension, kidney failure, liver steatosis, and many others.

1. Quality Sleep

An adult should sleep at least 7-8 hours each night.

It's also important to have a regular sleep that follows the circadian rhythm.

That's why you should rest at night for 7-8 hours.

While you sleep, your body activates a series of processes that repair and regenerate the body itself.

In addition, several studies prove the link between a lack of proper rest and the development of diseases such as diabetes, cancer, hypertension, and others.

2. Stop smoking

According to one study published in the National Library of Medicine, smoking causes 30% of all cancers.

But that's not all.

In fact, smoking stimulates the immune response and increases inflammation.

That's why, if you are a smoker, you should quit right now.

3. Exercising

Physical activity is crucial because it releases powerful anti-inflammatory substances: myokines.

One of these molecules is called Irisin and, in addition to lowering the inflammation in the body, it has many other important functions.

Among them, it helps lower blood sugar and cholesterol.

You don't need to toil in the gym every day or jog for hours.

As many doctors recommend, it's good enough to start with 30 minutes of light exercise – such as walking – 4 or 5 times a week.

4. Relieving stress

As I mentioned earlier, stress is one of the main causes of inflammation.

That's why you need to try and reduce it.

But how?

To start with, physical activity lends you a big helping hand in reducing stress levels.

You could also practice yoga or meditation.

5. Nutrition

As a recent Harvard University article puts it, "Doctors are learning that one of the best ways to reduce inflammation is not found in the medicine cabinet, but in the fridge".

But how can the right diet prevent or reverse inflammation?

Through the two mechanisms that I will shortly share with you.

So, if you want to learn how to organize your diet to activate the anti-inflammatory process – and which foods to favor or avoid – then read this section to the end.

4. The 2 principles of the anti-inflammatory diet

Now, let's dive into the thick of it.

As I told you earlier, nutrition plays a key

role in preventing and even reversing chronic inflammation.

In fact, the right diet can help you trigger a counter-inflammatory process.

You need to know that your diet should be based on two key principles:

- Reducing free radicals;
- Antioxidant intake.

Let me now explain why these two are key factors.

Let's start with the free radicals that I mentioned earlier.

Now I'll explain what they are and why you need to fight them.

Free radicals are waste products of our bodies.

They form through the body's normal reactions, such as the process by which we turn food into energy.

The problem with these substances is that they are unstable molecules.

What does that mean?

I'll try to explain it as plainly as possible.

These molecules are missing an electron – a sub-atomic particle.

I mean, it's quite like a car missing a wheel.

To regain their stability, they must "steal a wheel" from another molecule.

Therefore, during this process they remove an electron from elements such as DNA, making it unstable in turn.

As you may know, damaged DNA can cause mutations.

If the body fails to repair this damage, defective cells may develop, which could then give rise to a tumor.

That's why you need to reduce the production of free radicals.

The foods that produce the most of these substances are mainly refined carbohydrates, industrially processed foods, and unsaturated fats.

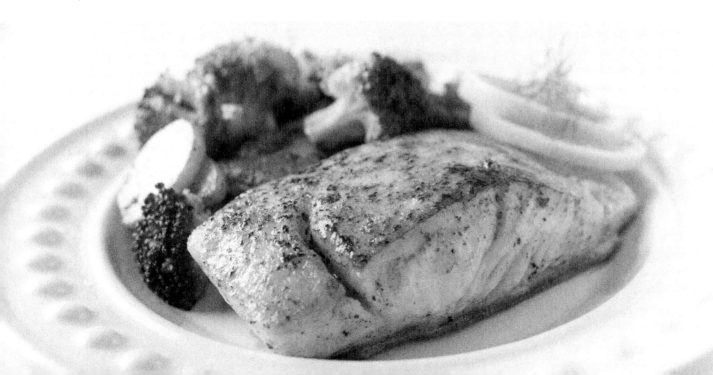

Therefore, I am soon going to give you a detailed list of which foods to reduce or eliminate from your diet.

Let us now concentrate on the second item: antioxidants.

Simply put, they are substances that can limit the damage caused by free radicals.

How do they do that?

In essence, they break the chain that triggers harmful molecules.

To do this, they interact with the "missing wheel" – that is, the missing electron.

They can stabilize the free radical, transforming it into a more stable compound.

At this point, the "fixed" waste is no longer as harmful as before and the body can eliminate it.

You should know that your body autonomously produces free radicals.

However, especially if your diet is imbalanced, the body alone cannot counteract the production of waste substances.

This is why eating the right foods can make a difference in preventing or reversing chronic inflammation.

The best foods to trigger this process are whole grains, good fats such as omega-3s, unprocessed foods, vitamins, and fiber from fruit and vegetables.

Therefore, a balanced diet should contain 4-5 units of fruit and vegetables every day.

In the last part, I will show you in detail what foods to include in your daily diet – and also the benefits they can provide.

But first, let me show you the 7 food types you should remove or reduce in your diet to fight inflammation.

5. The 7 food categories you should avoid

I'm now going to show you the types of foods of which you'll need to reduce your intake.

Obviously, this does not mean that you will have to permanently eliminate them from your diet.

However, several research projects and studies show how these foods increase the production of free radicals, promoting inflammatory processes.

Therefore, you need to keep their intake to a minimum, and only consume them as an occasional "treat".

Below I will list for you the "bad" foods for your health.

However, I'm not going to just provide a generic list.

In fact, I've decided to divide them by type and explain why they are harmful to your body.

1. Red Meat

For years now, studies have shown how red meat increases the risk of cancer.

But that's not all.

In fact, researchers at the University of Medicine in San Diego have discovered that this type of food also contains a particular molecule – not produced by the body.

Therefore, when we ingest this substance, our body does not recognize it – and attacks it, considering it to be an "external enemy", almost like a virus.

This ignites an inflammatory response, without you even noticing.

Therefore, you should reduce the consumption of red meat such as:

- Pork
- Beef

2. Sugar

As you certainly know well, sugars are infamous for their ability to raise blood sugar.

However, they are not only harmful to people with diabetes.

In fact, recent studies published in the National Library of Medicine show that their consumption is also associated with inflammation, chronic kidney disease, hepatic steatosis, and cancer.

But that's not all.

Sugars limit the anti-inflammatory power of omega-3s, the good fats that protect our health.

Therefore, you should reduce your intake of foods such as:

- Desserts
- Sweets
- Soda drinks
- Sweetened coffee and tea
- Maple and other syrups and honey

3. Refined Carbohydrates

Processed foods often contain refined carbohydrates.

The problem is that these foods also lack vitamins and fiber – elements that protect your health.

I mean, they are basically "empty" calories.

In addition, one study showed that adults who followed a diet rich in refined carbohydrates had a 2.9-fold higher risk of dying from an inflammatory disease.

Therefore, you should reduce your intake of foods such as:

- White bread
- Baked goods
- Snacks
- Pasta
- French fries
- Sweetened cereals

4. Saturated fats

Saturated fats have a dual negative role.

On the one hand, they increase bad cholesterol, thus exposing you to the risk of developing cardiovascular disease.

On the other hand, they promote inflammation.

Therefore, you should limit your consumption of:

- Butter
- Margarine
- Lard
- Fatty cheeses
- Desserts
- Fatty meat
- Fast foods

5. Cooking oils

Oil types widely used for cooking at home or in restaurants contain an excess of omega-6s, at the expense of omega-3s.

Some studies suggest that an unbalanced ratio of these substances may increase inflammation.

For this reason, avoid foods such as:

- Canola oil
- Corn oil
- Mayonnaise
- Sunflower seed oil
- Peanut oil

6. Processed meat

Processed meat often comes from animals fed with foods rich in omega-6s.

Therefore, the animal accumulates an excess of saturated and bad fats.

Additionally, various preservatives and chemicals are added to the meat itself.

Therefore, several studies show that the consumption of processed meat is linked to increased inflammation, heart disease, and cancer risk.

Reduce your intake of:

- Sausages
- Hamburgers
- Chicken nuggets

7. Alcohol

Moderate alcohol consumption should not cause problems for the body.

Indeed, research shows that it may even have some benefits.

However, excessive alcohol intake may boost inflammation.

That's why you should limit alcohol consumption.

Finally, it might seem obvious but of course you should steer clear of any foods you have an intolerance or allergy to.

Maybe you are still unaware of being oversensitive to gluten or lactose.

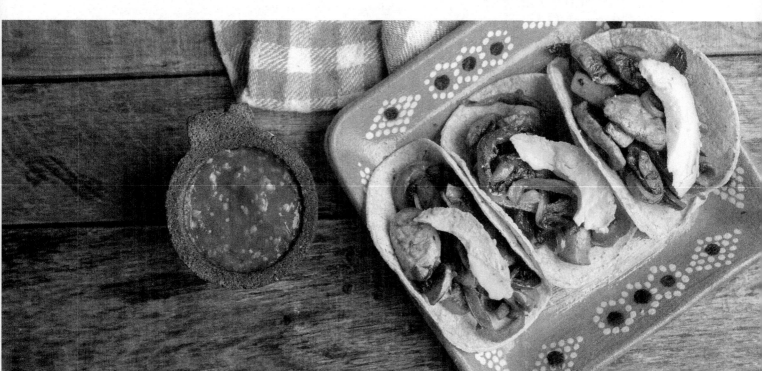

So, if you feel bloated after eating a plate of pasta, pizza, or cheese, or find you have trouble digesting or discomfort after certain meals, then I would definitely recommend testing to find out if you are intolerant. You might be surprised at the results, and it could be a very simple fix to eliminate those ingredients and transform your health.

Well, so far I have shown you which foods are "bad" for your health.

Next, I will reveal the anti-inflammatory foods that you should include in your diet.

6. 16 powerful anti-inflammatory foods

I want to introduce you to the best foods you should include in your diet to prevent or reverse inflammation.

Again, I won't just provide a simple list.

Instead, I will give you a detailed list of the foods – and benefits they can offer.

Obviously, it does not mean that your diet should only consist of these foods.

However, my advice is that you should bear them in mind and if possible consume them more often than you are doing now.

So, here are the 16 foods you should include in your diet.

1. Berries

Berries are rich in fiber, vitamins, and minerals.

They also contain powerful antioxidants, as recent studies show.

Therefore, they play a crucial role against free radicals and thus help to combat inflammation.

So, in your diet you might include:

- Strawberries
- Blueberries
- Raspberries
- Blackberries

2. Oily fish

Fatty fish you can eat includes:

- Salmon
- Sardines
- Herring
- Mackerel.

These types of fish have a high content of omega-3s.

As several studies published in the National Library of Medicine show, these substances are very powerful anti-inflammatory agents.

3. Broccoli

Broccoli is rich in vitamin C, minerals, and fiber.

They also contain an important antioxidant that helps fight inflammation.

4. Avocado

Avocado is rich in potassium, magnesium, and vitamins.

It is also a source of good fats, which preserve the health of the heart.

It also contains very useful anti-inflammatory substances for the body.

5. Green tea

This drink has several benefits for the human body.

To begin with, recent studies show how green tea helps reduce the risk of Alzheimer's, heart problems, and cancer.

It also has a powerful antioxidant effect, so it helps fight inflammation.

You might want to consider including it in your breakfast menu.

6. Bell Peppers

These vegetables are rich in vitamin C and minerals.

They also contain several antioxidants to counteract the inflammatory process.

7. Mushrooms

There are countless varieties of mushrooms.

They are rich in selenium and vitamin B.

You can enjoy them both raw and cooked.

However, according to one study, their antioxidant power is greater after cooking.

8. Grapes

Grapes have very interesting properties; therefore, they have been the object of several studies.

Thanks to their antioxidant, not only do they help reduce the risk of diabetes, Alzheimer's, and vision disorders, but it also has excellent anti-inflammatory properties.

9. Turmeric

In recent years, researchers have conducted many studies on turmeric.

It contains curcumin, a powerful anti-inflammatory substance.

That's why you may want to use it to season your dishes.

Besides being important for your health, it will also help you give a spicy touch to your recipes.

10. Extra virgin olive oil (EVO)

Compared to other cooking oils, extra virgin olive oil has many more beneficial effects.

In one study, people who consumed it on a daily basis showed a reduction in inflammation.

In fact, EVO oil doesn't just contain good fats for your heart.

It is also rich in anti-inflammatory substances that help prevent diseases such as cancer.

11. Dark chocolate

You should choose chocolate with at least 70% cocoa.

Indeed, dark chocolate is rich in flavonoids – powerful substances that fight inflammation.

But that's not all.

In fact, in one study, people who consumed cocoa flavonoids showed an improvement in vascular function in just 2 weeks.

12. Tomatoes

They are rich in vitamin C.

They also contain lycopene, a very powerful antioxidant that counteracts the inflammatory processes typical of various types of cancer.

13. Cherries

In addition to being delicious, they are also rich in antioxidants.

This is why you may want to include them in your diet, perhaps as snacks or at breakfast.

14. Leafy greens

Green leafy vegetables, such as spinach or rocket, are rich in antioxidants.

They also contain vitamins, minerals, and fiber.

Therefore, you should always include a portion of vegetables at lunch and dinner.

15. Nuts

They are rich in vitamins A and K.

They also contain vitamin E, one of the most powerful antioxidants.

This is why nuts have a strong anti-inflammatory effect.

Finally, they are rich in good fats such as omega-3s, which are important for heart health.

So, your daily diet might include:

- Walnuts
- Almonds
- Pistachios
- Hazelnuts

Note that peanuts are not actually tree-nuts, so are not included in this list.

16. Wholegrain cereals

Unlike refined cereals, whole grains are rich in fiber and nutrients.

They also have a lower glycemic index.

This is why they don't cause your blood sugar to raise so steeply and they reduce the risk of diabetes.

Hence, in your diet you could include:

- Brown rice and wholegrain pasta
- Wholemeal bread
- Oats
- Barley
- Spelt
- Whole wheat

Conclusion

Having told you the foods that can help you prevent inflammation, we have now reached the end of this section.

By now you should have a clearer idea of what chronic inflammation is, what its causes are, and what remedies there are to reverse the inflammatory process.

In the last part, I showed you the foods you may want to include in your diet to take better care of your body.

Now you are ready to discover 150 delicious recipes that will help you prevent chronic inflammation – or reverse it – in just 3 months.

Thanks to these recipes, you can combine different options and enjoy a different menu every day, for more than 1,000 days.

Wondering how that's possible?

Most people have breakfast, snack and two main meals a day.

The choice is up to you of course, but let's take that as an example, even keeping it more simple by assuming you have your routine same breakfast each day.

I have given you 41 fish, meat and poultry dishes and 39 vegetarian, salad and soup recipes. Just going through my choices one by one in order choosing the vegetarian, salad or soup options for lunch and a fish, meat or poultry recipe for dinner means you won't get the same combination for a second time until 1600 days have passed!!

It's really that easy to give yourself an interesting healthy and varied diet.

And even more, I have given you 12 sauces that you can add to simple steamed fish fillets or vegetables, salads and a small portion of wholegrain pasta for example, which means you can vary your options even more.

And I also have given you 10 side dishes that you can combine with your other recipe choices. At this point the possibilities really are endless!

So, you can see that even if there are some ingredients that you don't enjoy, you can easily make choices tailored to you and have a different menu combination to enjoy for over 1,000 days.

Now, I leave it to you to discover these tasty recipes, thanks to which you can take care of your own and your loved ones' health, as well as enjoying food together.

I decided to include some dessert recipes in this book because we all need a treat every once in a while!

However please remember that in a low calories regime you have to consume desserts ONLY as a special treat, say, on special occasions. I would suggest once a month is reasonable but if you have any health concerns remember to get advice from your doctor.

Regarding red meat, I suggest to reduce consumption to once per week to maximize the benefits of this diet and reduce inflammation.

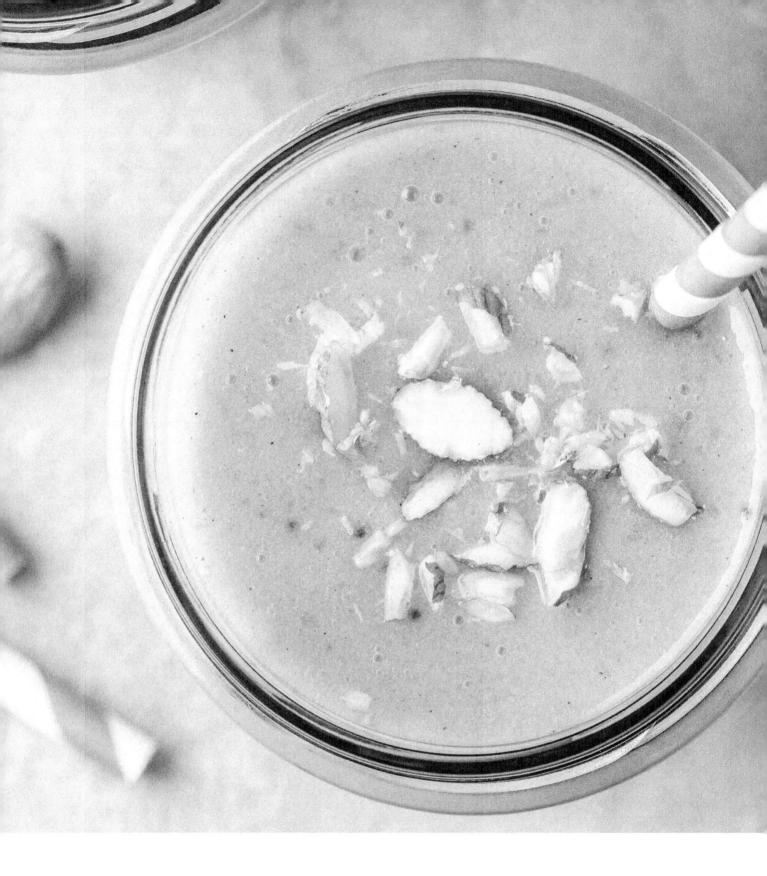

GREEN VANILLA SMOOTHIE

10 minutes

0 minutes

1

INGREDIENTS

- 1 banana, cut into chunks
- 1 cup of grapes
- 1 tub (6 oz.) vanilla yogurt
- ½ apple, cored and chopped
- 1 ½ cups fresh spinach leaves

DIRECTIONS

1. Add everything to a blender jug.
2. Cover the jug tightly.
3. Blend until smooth. Serve and enjoy!

NUTRITION

Calories: 480 Kcal; Protein: 8 g; Carbohydrates: 105 g; Fat: 4 g

PURPLE FRUIT SMOOTHIE

10 minutes

0 minutes

1

INGREDIENTS

- 2 bananas, frozen, cut into chunks
- ½ cup blueberries, frozen
- 1 cup orange juice
- 1 tbsp honey, optional
- 1 tsp vanilla extract, optional

DIRECTIONS

1. Add everything to a blender jug.
2. Cover the jug tightly.
3. Blend until smooth. Serve and enjoy!

NUTRITION

Calories: 374 Kcal; Protein: 4 g; Carbohydrates: 84 g; Fat: 1 g

Vanilla Avocado Smoothie

INGREDIENTS

- 1 ripe avocado, halved and pitted
- 1 cup almond milk
- ½ cup vanilla yogurt
- 3 tbsp honey
- 8 ice cubes

DIRECTIONS

1. Add everything to a blender jug.
2. Cover the jug tightly
3. Blend until smooth. Serve and enjoy!

NUTRITION

Calories: 510 Kcal; Protein: 8 g; Carbohydrates: 56 g; Fat: 28 g

3

10 minutes

0 minutes

1

TRIPLE FRUIT SMOOTHIE

INGREDIENTS

- 1 kiwi, sliced
- 1 banana, peeled and chopped
- ½ cup blueberries
- 1 cup strawberries
- 1 cup ice cubes
- ½ cup orange juice
- 1 container (8 oz.) of peach yogurt

DIRECTIONS

1. Add everything to a blender jug.
2. Cover the jug tightly
3. Blend until smooth. Serve and enjoy!

NUTRITION

Calories: 496 Kcal; Protein: 12 g; Carbohydrates: 109 g; Fat: 2 g

4

10 minutes

0 minutes

1

PEACH MAPLE SMOOTHIE

10 minutes

0 minutes

1

INGREDIENTS

- 4 large peaches, peeled and chopped
- 2 tbsp maple syrup
- 1 cup fat-free yogurt
- 1 cup of ice

DIRECTIONS

1. Add everything to a blender jug.
2. Cover the jug tightly.
3. Blend until smooth. Serve and enjoy!

NUTRITION

Calories: 197 Kcal; Protein: 8 g; Carbohydrates: 39 g; Fat: 0 g

PINK CALIFORNIA SMOOTHIE

10 minutes

0 minutes

1

INGREDIENTS

- 7 large strawberries
- 1 container (8 oz.) of lemon yogurt
- ⅓ cup orange juice

DIRECTIONS

1. Add everything to a blender jug.
2. Cover the jug tightly.
3. Blend until smooth. Serve and enjoy!

NUTRITION

Calories: 366 Kcal; Protein: 7 g; Carbohydrates: 77 g; Fat: 4 g

MANGO AND GINGER INFUSED WATER

INGREDIENTS

- 1 cup fresh mango, chopped
- 2" piece ginger, peeled, cubed
- Water, to cover ingredients

DIRECTIONS

1. Place ingredients in the mesh steamer basket.
2. Place the basket in the instant pot.
3. Add water to cover contents.
4. Lock the lid. Cook on HIGH pressure for 5 minutes.
5. Once done, release pressure quickly.
6. Remove steamer basket. Discard cooked produce.
7. Allow flavored water to cool. Chill completely. Serve.

5 minutes

5 minutes

4

NUTRITION

Calories: 166 Kcal; Protein: 3 g; Carbohydrates: 38 g; Fat: 1 g

PEACH AND RASPBERRY LEMONADE

INGREDIENTS

- 1 cup fresh peaches, chopped
- ½ cup fresh raspberries
- Zest and juice of 1 lemon
- Water, to cover ingredients

DIRECTIONS

1. Place ingredients in a mesh basket for instant pot. Place in pot.
2. Add water to barely cover the fruit.
3. Lock the lid. Cook on HIGH pressure for 5 minutes.
4. Once done, release pressure quickly.
5. Remove steamer basket. Discard cooked produce.
6. Allow flavored water to cool. Chill completely before serving.

5 minutes

5 minutes

4

NUTRITION

Calories: 105 Kcal; Protein: 1 g; Carbohydrates: 24 g; Fat: 0 g

SWEET CRANBERRY JUICE

5 minutes

8 minutes

4

INGREDIENTS

- 4 cups fresh cranberries
- 1 cinnamon stick
- 1-gallon filtered water
- ½ cup honey
- Juice of 1 lemon

DIRECTIONS

1. Add cranberries, ½ of water, and cinnamon stick to the instant pot.
2. Lock the lid. Cook on HIGH pressure for 8 minutes.
3. Release pressure naturally.
4. Once cool, strain the liquid. Add remaining water.
5. Stir in honey and lemon. Cool completely.
6. Chill before serving.

NUTRITION

Calories: 236 Kcal; Protein: 2 g; Carbohydrates: 55 g; Fat: 1 g

---

VANILLA TURMERIC ORANGE JUICE

5 minutes

0 minutes

2

INGREDIENTS

- 6 oranges, peeled, separated into segments, deseeded
- 2 tsp vanilla extract
- ½ tsp turmeric powder
- 2 cups unsweetened almond milk
- 1 tsp cinnamon, ground
- Pepper, to taste

DIRECTIONS

1. Juice the oranges. Add the rest of the ingredients.
2. Pour into glasses and serve.

NUTRITION

Calories: 282 Kcal; Protein: 6.4 g; Carbohydrates: 50 g; Fat: 7 g

CUCUMBER KIWI GREEN SMOOTHIE

INGREDIENTS

- 2 ripe kiwi fruit
- 1 cup cucumber, seedless, chopped
- 1 cup coconut water
- 6 to 8 ice cubes
- ¼ cup coconut milk, canned
- 2 tbsp fresh cilantro, chopped

DIRECTIONS

1. Combine the smoothie ingredients in your high-speed blender.
2. Pulse a few times to cut them up.
3. Blend the mixture on the highest speed setting for 30 to 60 seconds.
4. Pour your finished smoothie into glasses and drink.

5 minutes

0 minutes

NUTRITION

Calories: 194 Kcal; Protein: 5 g; Carbohydrates: 18 g; Fat: 12 g

2

TROPICAL PINEAPPLE KIWI SMOOTHIE

INGREDIENTS

- 1 ½ cups pineapple, frozen
- 1 ripe kiwi; peeled and chopped
- 1 cup full-fat coconut milk, canned
- 6 to 8 ice cubes
- 1 tsp spirulina powder
- 3 tsp lime juice

DIRECTIONS

1. Combine the smoothie ingredients in your high-speed blender.
2. Pulse a few times to cut them up.
3. Blend the mixture on the highest speed setting.
4. Pour your finished smoothie into glasses and drink.

5 minutes

0 minutes

NUTRITION

Calories: 300 Kcal; Protein: 4 g; Carbohydrates: 44 g; Fat: 10 g

2

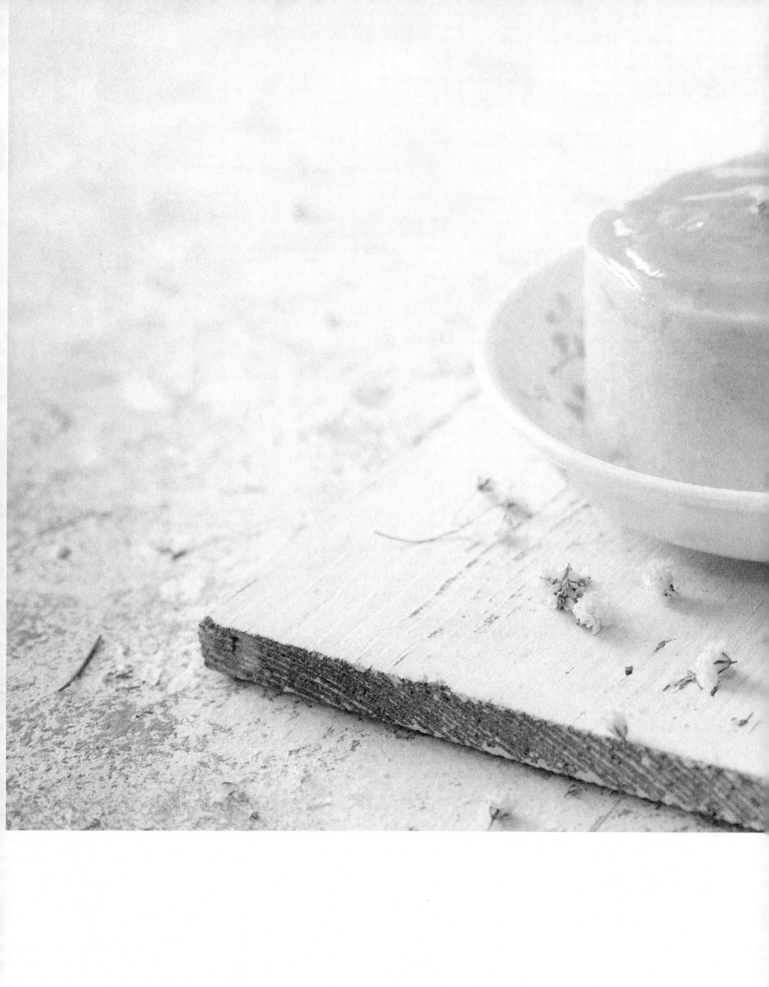

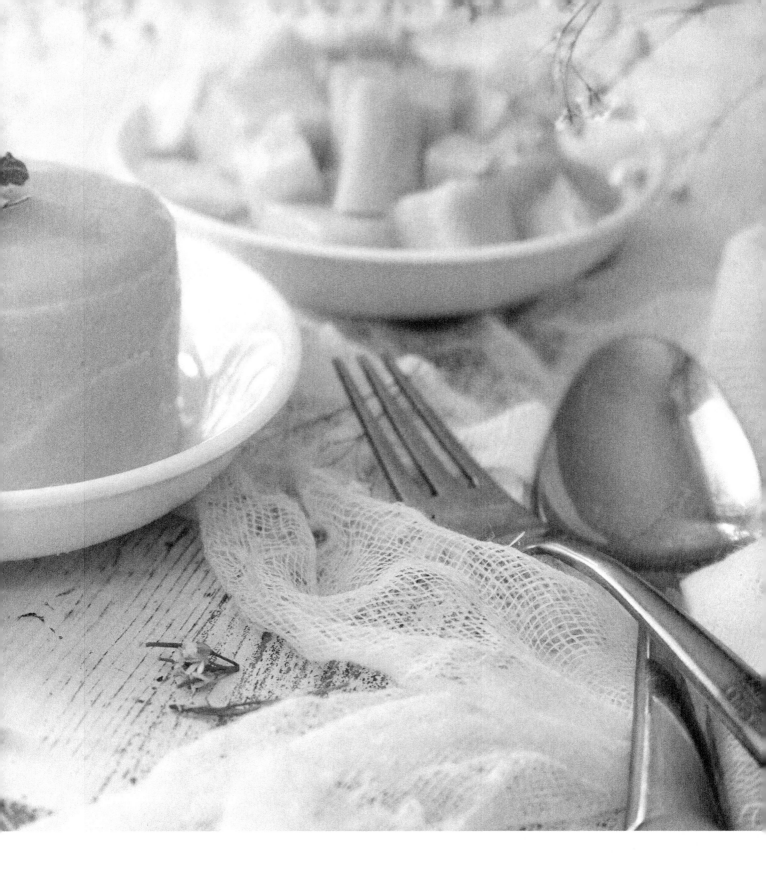

CHAPTER 2
FRUIT RECIPES

MANGO MUG CAKE

5 minutes

10 minutes

2

INGREDIENTS

- 1 medium-sized mango, peeled and diced
- 2 eggs
- 1 tsp vanilla
- ¼ tsp nutmeg, grated
- 1 tbsp cocoa powder
- 2 tbsp honey
- ½ cup coconut flour

DIRECTIONS

1. Combine the coconut flour, eggs, honey, vanilla, nutmeg, and cocoa powder in 2 lightly greased mugs.
2. Then, add 1 cup of water and a metal trivet to the Instant Pot. Lower the uncovered mugs onto the trivet.
3. Secure the lid. Choose the "Manual" mode and High pressure; cook for 10 minutes. Once cooking is complete, use a quick pressure release; carefully remove the lid.
4. Top with diced mango and serve chilled. Enjoy!

NUTRITION

Calories: 465 Kcal; Protein: 21 g; Carbohydrates:47 g; Fat: 19 g

---

HONEY STEWED APPLES

5 minutes

5 minutes

4

INGREDIENTS

- 2 tbsp honey
- 1 tsp cinnamon, ground
- ½ tsp cloves, ground
- 4 apples

DIRECTIONS

1. Add all ingredients to the inner pot. Now, pour in ⅓ cup of water.
2. Secure the lid. Choose the "Manual" mode and cook for 2 minutes at high pressure. Once cooking is complete, use a quick pressure release; carefully remove the lid.
3. Serve in individual bowls. Bon appétit!

NUTRITION

Calories: 458 Kcal; Protein: 2 g; Carbohydrates: 121 g; Fat: 2 g

ORANGE BUTTERSCOTCH PUDDING

INGREDIENTS

- 4 caramels
- 2 eggs, well-beaten
- ¼ cup orange juice, freshly squeezed
- ⅓ cup sugar
- 1 cup cake flour
- ½ tsp baking powder
- ¼ cup milk
- 1 stick of butter, melted
- ½ tsp vanilla essence

Sauce:

- ½ cup golden syrup
- 2 tsp corn flour
- 1 cup boiling water

DIRECTIONS

1. Melt the butter and milk in the microwave. Whisk in the eggs, vanilla, and sugar. After that, stir in the flour, baking powder, and orange juice.
2. Lastly, add the caramels and stir until everything is well combined and melted.
3. Divide between the 4 jars. Add 1 ½ cup of water and a metal trivet to the bottom of the Instant Pot. Lower the jars onto the trivet.
4. To make the sauce, whisk the boiling water, corn flour, and golden syrup until everything is well combined. Pour the sauce into each jar.
5. Secure the lid. Choose the "Steam" mode and cook for 15 minutes under high pressure. Once cooking is complete, use a natural pressure release; carefully remove the lid. Enjoy!

10 minutes

15 minutes

4

NUTRITION

Calories: 800 Kcal; Protein: 37 g; Carbohydrates: 120 g; Fat: 35 g

RUBY PEARS DELIGHT

INGREDIENTS

- 4 pears
- 26 oz. grape juice
- 11 oz. currant jelly
- 2 garlic cloves
- Juice and zest of 1 lemon
- 4 peppercorns
- 2 rosemary sprigs
- ½ vanilla bean

DIRECTIONS

1. Pour the jelly and grape juice into your instant pot and mix with lemon zest and juice.
2. In the mix, dip each pear and wrap them in a clean tin foil and place them orderly in the steamer basket of your instant pot.
3. Combine peppercorns, rosemary, garlic cloves, and vanilla bean into the juice mixture.
4. Seal the lid and cook at High for 10 minutes.
5. Release the pressure quickly, and carefully open the lid; bring out the pears, remove wrappers and arrange them on plates. Serve when cold with toppings of cooking juice.

10 minutes

10 minutes

4

NUTRITION

Calories: 980 Kcal; Protein: 4 g; Carbohydrates: 200 g; Fat: 1 g

MIXED BERRY AND ORANGE COMPOTE

15 minutes

15 minutes

4

INGREDIENTS

- ½-lb. strawberries
- 1 tbsp orange juice
- ¼ tsp cloves, ground
- ½ cup brown sugar
- 1 vanilla bean
- 1-lb. blueberries
- ½-lb. blackberries

DIRECTIONS

1. Place your berries in the inner pot. Add the sugar and let sit for 15 minutes. Add in the orange juice, ground cloves, and vanilla bean.
2. Secure the lid. Choose the "Manual" mode and cook for 2 minutes at high pressure. Once cooking is complete, use a natural pressure release for 10 minutes; carefully remove the lid.
3. As your compote cools, it will thicken. Bon appétit!

NUTRITION

Calories: 697 Kcal; Protein: 8 g; Carbohydrates: 120 g; Fat: 3 g

STREUSELKUCHEN WITH PEACHES

10 minutes

20 minutes

6

INGREDIENTS

- 1 cup oats, rolled
- 1 tsp vanilla extract
- ⅓ cup orange juice
- 4 tbsp raisins
- 2 tbsp honey
- 4 tbsp butter
- 4 tbsp all-purpose flour
- A pinch of nutmeg, grated
- ½ tsp cardamom, ground
- A pinch of salt
- 1 tsp cinnamon, ground
- 6 peaches, pitted and chopped
- ⅓ cup brown sugar

DIRECTIONS

1. Place the peaches on the bottom of the inner pot. Sprinkle with cardamom, cinnamon, and vanilla. Top with orange juice, honey, and raisins.
2. In a mixing bowl, whisk together the butter, oats, flour, brown sugar, nutmeg, and salt. Drop a spoonful on top of the peaches.
3. Secure the lid. Choose the "Manual" mode and cook for 8 minutes at high pressure. Once cooking is complete, use a natural pressure release for 10 minutes; carefully remove the lid. Bon appétit!

NUTRITION

Calories: 989 Kcal; Protein: 25 g; Carbohydrates: 200 g; Fat: 15 g

AVOCADO AND SAUERKRAUT

INGREDIENTS

- ¼ avocado, pitted and mashed
- 1 tsp homemade sauerkraut
- 1 pinch of Celtic Sea salt

DIRECTIONS

1. Slice the avocado and mash with the sauerkraut.
2. Season with salt and enjoy right away.

NUTRITION

Calories: 232 Kcal; Protein: 3 g; Carbohydrates: 2 g; Fat: 23 g

5 minutes

0 minutes

1

DELICIOUS COCONUT MACAROONS

INGREDIENTS

- 1 tbsp raw cocoa powder
- 3 dates, pitted
- 2 tsp vanilla extract
- ¼ cup raisins
- 6 egg whites
- 2 cups coconut, unsweetened and shredded
- ⅛ tsp sea salt

DIRECTIONS

1. Preheat the oven to 350°F/176°C.
2. Combine all ingredients in the bowl.
3. Line the baking tray with parchment paper.
4. Place 1 tbsp of dough on the baking tray. Press down to flatten.
5. Bake in preheated oven for around 15 minutes or until golden.
6. Serve and enjoy.

NUTRITION

Calories: 500 Kcal; Protein: 20 g; Carbohydrates: 50 g; Fat: 16 g

5 minutes

30 minutes

6

21

10 minutes

3 minutes

6

PEACH COMPOTE

INGREDIENTS

- 8 peaches, pitted and chopped
- 6 tbsp sugar
- 1 tsp cinnamon, ground
- 1 tsp vanilla extract
- 1 vanilla bean, scraped
- 2 tbsp Grape Nuts cereal

DIRECTIONS

1. Put the peaches into the Instant Pot and mix with the sugar, cinnamon, vanilla bean, and vanilla extract. Stir well, cover the Instant Pot and cook on the Manual setting for 3 minutes.
2. Release the pressure for 10 minutes, add the cereal, stir well, transfer the compote to bowls, and serve.

NUTRITION

Calories: 496 Kcal; Protein: 10 g; Carbohydrates: 121 g; Fat: 3 g

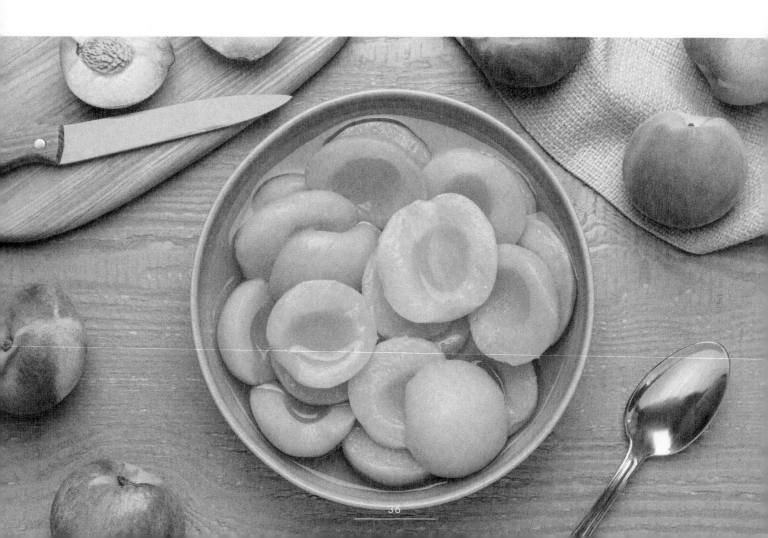

PISTACHIO AND FRUITS

INGREDIENTS

- ½ cup apricots, dried and chopped
- ¼ cup cranberries, dried
- ½ tsp cinnamon
- ¼ tsp allspice
- ¼ tsp nutmeg, ground
- 1 ¼ cups pistachios, unsalted and roasted
- 2 tsp sugar

DIRECTIONS

1. Start by heating the oven to a temperature of around 345°F.
2. Using a tray, place the pistachios and bake for seven minutes. Allow the pistachio to cool afterward.
3. Combine all ingredients in a container.
4. Once everything is combined well, the food is ready to serve.

NUTRITION

Calories: 373 Kcal; Protein: 8 g; Carbohydrates: 60 g; Fat: 14 g

5 minutes

7 minutes

12

AVOCADO SORBET

INGREDIENTS

- ¼ cup sugar
- 1 cup of water
- 1 tsp lime zest, grated
- 1 tbsp honey
- 2 ripe avocados, pitted and skin removed
- 2 tbsp lime juice

DIRECTIONS

1. Combine the sugar and water in a small pan over medium flame. Continue until the sugar dissolves completely, and then remove from the flame.
2. Place the avocados in the food processor. Add the sugar and water mix along with the honey, lime zest, and lime juice into the food processor.
3. Process until you reach a smooth consistency.
4. Place the mix into a baking pan and cover with foil. Place the mix into the freezer until completely frozen.
5. Upon serving, process the food in the food processor until you reach a smooth consistency.

NUTRITION

Calories: 534 Kcal; Protein: 6 g; Carbohydrates: 38 g; Fat: 43 g

5 minutes

10 minutes

4

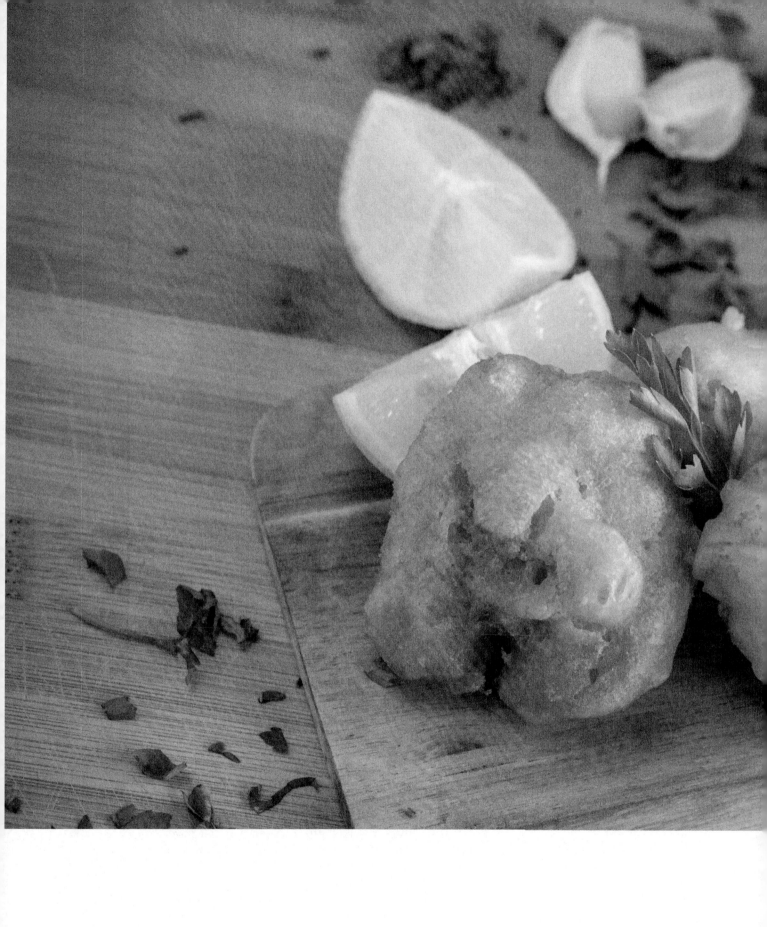

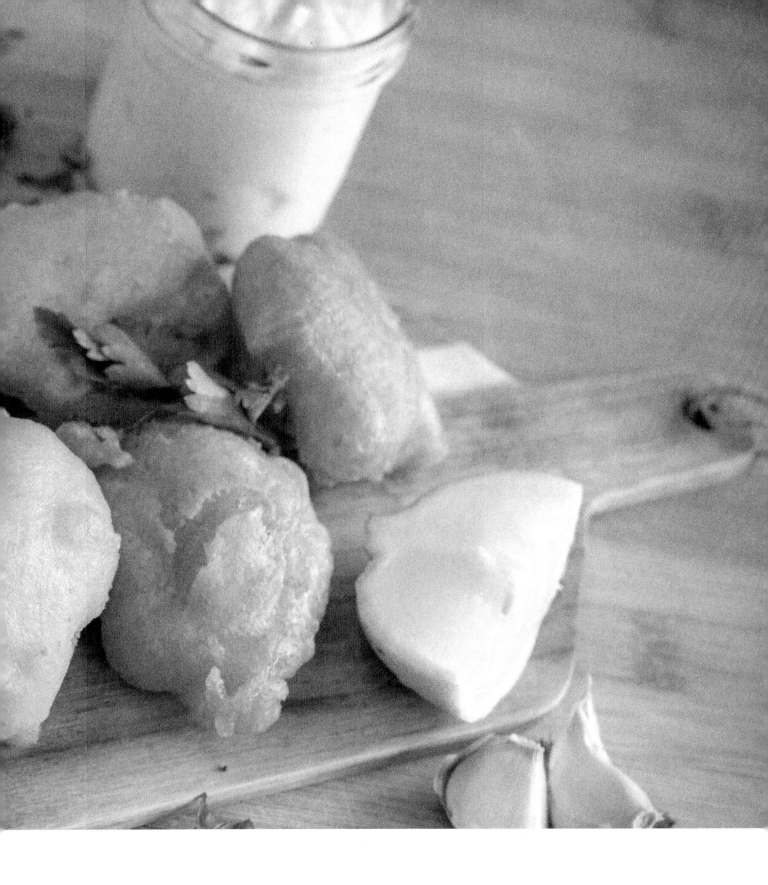

20 minutes

30 minutes

4

Pan-Seared Haddock with Beets

INGREDIENTS

- 8 beets, peeled and cut into 8hs
- 2 shallots, thinly sliced
- 1 tsp bottled garlic, minced
- 2 tbsp olive oil, divided
- 2 tbsp apple cider vinegar
- 1 tsp fresh thyme, chopped
- Pinch sea salt
- 4 (5-oz. / 142-g) haddock fillets, patted dry

DIRECTIONS

1. Preheat the oven to 400°F (205°C).
2. In a medium bowl, toss together the beets, shallots, garlic, and 1 tbsp of olive oil until well coated. Spread the beet mixture in a 9-x-13" baking dish. Roast for about 30 minutes, or until the vegetables are caramelized and tender.
3. Remove the beets from the oven and stir in the cider vinegar, thyme, and sea salt.
4. While the beets are roasting, place a large skillet over medium-high heat and add the remaining 1 tbsp of olive oil.
5. Panfry the fish for about 15 minutes, turning once, until it flakes when pressed with a fork. Serve the fish with a generous scoop of roasted beets.

Storage: Store in an airtight container in the fridge for up to 4 days or in the freezer for up to 1 month.

Reheat: Microwave, covered, until the desired temperature is reached.

NUTRITION

Calories: 342 Kcal; Protein: 30 g; Carbohydrates: 21 g; Fat: 9 g

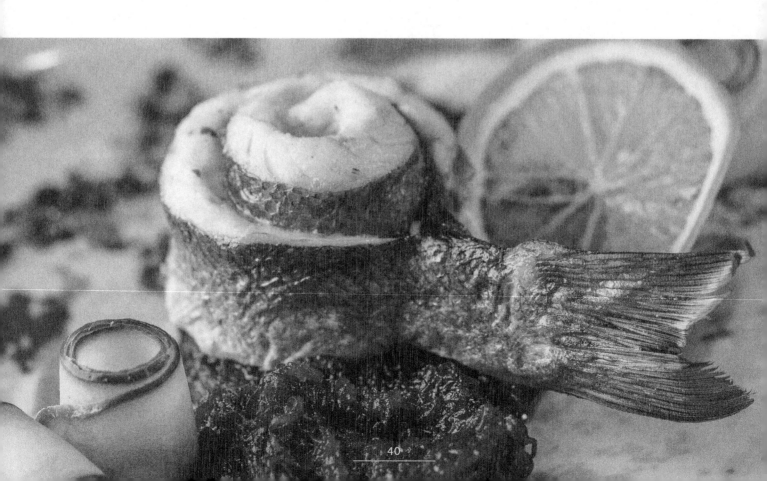

FISH TACO SALAD WITH STRAWBERRY AVOCADO SALSA

INGREDIENTS

For the salsa:

- 2 strawberries, hulled and diced
- ½ small shallot, diced
- 2 tbsp fresh cilantro, finely chopped
- 2 tbsp lime juice, freshly squeezed
- 1 tsp cayenne pepper
- ½ avocado, diced
- 2 tbsp black beans, canned, rinsed, and drained
- 1 green onion, thinly sliced
- ½ tsp ginger, finely chopped, peeled
- ¼ tsp sea salt

For the fish:

- 1 tsp agave nectar
- 2 cups arugula
- 1 tbsp extra-virgin olive oil or avocado oil
- ½ tbsp lime juice, freshly squeezed
- 1 lb. light fish (halibut, cod, or red snapper), cut into 2 fillets
- ¼ tsp black pepper, freshly ground
- ½ tsp sea salt

DIRECTIONS

1. Preheat the grill, whether it's gas or charcoal.
2. To create the salsa, add the avocado, beans, strawberries, shallot, cilantro, green onions, salt, cayenne pepper, ginger, and lime juice in a medium mixing cup. Put aside after mixing until all of the components are well combined.
3. To render the salad, whisk together the agave, oil, and lime juice in a small bowl. Toss the arugula with the vinaigrette in a big mixing bowl.
4. Season the fish fillets with pepper and salt. Grill the fish for around 7 to 9 minutes over direct high heat, flipping once during cooking. The fish should be translucent and quickly flake.
5. Place 1 cup of arugula salad on each plate to eat. Cover each salad with a fillet and a heaping spoonful of salsa.

20 minutes

10 minutes

2

NUTRITION

Calories: 431 Kcal; Protein: 12 g; Carbohydrates: 50 g; Fat: 22 g

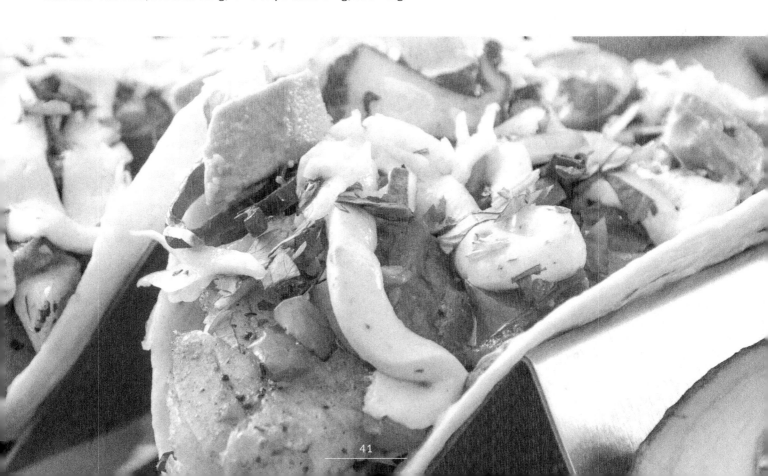

26

10 minutes

20 minutes

4

SHRIMP MUSHROOM SQUASH

INGREDIENTS

- 2 tbsp hemp seeds
- 2 tbsp olive oil
- 1 lb. shrimp, peeled and deveined
- ¼ cup coconut aminos
- 2 tbsp raw honey
- 2 tsp sesame oil
- 1 yellow onion, chopped
- 4 oz. shiitake mushrooms, (cut into slices)
- 2 garlic cloves, minced
- 1 red bell pepper, (cut into slices)
- 1 yellow squash, peeled and cubed
- 2 cups chard, chopped

DIRECTIONS

1. In a bowl (medium size), mix the aminos, honey, sesame oil, and hemp seeds.
2. In a skillet (you can also use a saucepan); heat the oil over the medium stove flame.
3. Add the onions, stir the mixture and cook while stirring for about 2-3 minutes until softened.
4. Add the bell pepper, squash, mushrooms, and garlic, and stir-cook for 5 minutes.
5. Add the shrimp and aminos mix; stir-cook for 4 minutes more.
6. Add the chard, toss; add into serving bowls and serve.

NUTRITION

Calories: 569 Kcal; Protein: 91 g; Carbohydrates: 50 g; Fat: 36 g

---

27

10 minutes

30 minutes

2

SPINACH SEA BASS LUNCH

INGREDIENTS

- 2 sea bass fillets, boneless
- 2 shallots, chopped
- Juice of ½ lemon
- 1 garlic clove, minced
- 5 cherry tomatoes, halved
- 1 tbsp parsley, chopped
- 1 tbsp olive oil
- 8 oz. baby spinach

DIRECTIONS

1. Preheat an oven to 450°F. Grease a baking dish with cooking spray.
2. Add the fish, tomatoes, parsley, and garlic, and drizzle the lemon juice.
3. Cover the dish and bake for 12–15 minutes and add in serving plates.
4. In a skillet (you can also use a saucepan); heat the oil over the medium stove flame.
5. Add the shallots, stir the mixture and cook while stirring for about 1-2 minutes until softened.
6. Add the spinach, stir, and cook for 4-5 minutes more. Add with the fish and serve warm.

NUTRITION

Calories: 214 Kcal; Protein: 26 g; Carbohydrates: 11 g; Fat: 9 g

GARLIC COD MEAL

INGREDIENTS

- 2 tbsp olive oil
- 2 tbsp tarragon, chopped
- ¼ cup parsley, chopped
- 4 cod fillets, skinless
- 2 garlic cloves, minced
- 1 yellow onion, chopped
- Black pepper, ground, and salt, to taste
- Juice of 1 lemon
- 1 lemon, (cut into slices)
- 1 tbsp thyme, chopped
- 4 cups of water

DIRECTIONS

1. In a skillet (you can also use a saucepan); heat the oil over the medium stove flame.
2. Add the onions, and garlic, stir the mixture, and cook while stirring for about 2–3 minutes until softened.
3. Add the salt, pepper, tarragon, parsley, thyme, water, lemon juice, and lemon slices.
4. Boil the mix; add the cod, cook for 12-15 minutes, and drain the liquid.
5. Serve with a side salad.

NUTRITION

Calories: 251 Kcal; Protein: 16 g; Carbohydrates: 19 g; Fat: 14 g

28

5 minutes

35 minutes

4

COD CUCUMBER DELIGHT

INGREDIENTS

- 1 tbsp capers, drained
- 4 tbsp + 1 tsp olive oil
- 4 cod fillets, skinless and boneless
- 2 tbsp mustard
- 1 tbsp tarragon, chopped
- Black pepper, ground, and salt, to the taste
- 2 cups lettuce leaves, torn
- 1 small red onion, (cut into slices)
- 1 small cucumber, (cut into slices)
- 2 tbsp lemon juice
- 2 tbsp water

DIRECTIONS

1. In a bowl (medium size), mix the mustard with 2 tbsp olive oil, tarragon, capers, and water, whisk well and set aside.
2. In a skillet (you can also use a saucepan); heat 1 tsp oil over the medium stove flame.
3. Add the fish, pepper, salt, and cook, while stirring, until well cooked and softened on both sides.
4. In a bowl (medium size), mix the cucumber, onion, lettuce, lemon juice, 2 tbsp olive oil, salt, and pepper.
5. Arrange the cod on serving plates, and top with the tarragon sauce.
6. Serve with the cucumber salad.

NUTRITION

Calories: 521 Kcal; Protein: 57 g; Carbohydrates: 21 g; Fat: 19 g

29

10 minutes

25 minutes

4

OREGANO LETTUCE SHRIMP

5 minutes

25 minutes

4

INGREDIENTS

- 3 tbsp dill, chopped
- 1 tbsp oregano, chopped
- 2 garlic cloves, chopped
- 1 lb. shrimp, deveined and peeled
- 2 tsp olive oil
- 6 tbsp lemon juice
- Black pepper, ground, and salt, to taste
- 2 cucumbers, (cut into slices)
- 1 red onion, (cut into slices)
- ¾ cup coconut cream
- ½ lb. cherry tomatoes
- 8 lettuce leaves

DIRECTIONS

1. In a bowl (medium size), combine the shrimp, 1 tbsp oregano, 2 tbsp lemon juice, 1 tbsp dill, and 1 tsp oil. Set aside for 10 minutes.
2. In another bowl, mix 1 tbsp dill, half of the garlic, ¼ cup coconut cream, 2 tbsp lemon juice, cucumber, salt, and pepper. Combine well.
3. In another bowl, mix the rest of the lemon juice, ½ cup of cream, the rest of the garlic, and the rest of the dill.
4. In a bowl (medium size), mix the tomatoes with onion and 1 tsp olive oil.
5. Heat a grill over medium-high heat, grill tomato mix, and shrimp mix for 5 minutes.
6. Add them to serving plates, and add the cucumber salad, lettuce leaves, and other ingredients on top.

NUTRITION

Calories: 569 Kcal; Protein: 50 g; Carbohydrates: 27 g; Fat: 19 g

MEXICAN PEPPER SALMON

5 minutes

25 minutes

4

INGREDIENTS

- 1 garlic clove, minced
- 1 tsp sweet paprika
- 4 medium salmon fillets, boneless
- 2 tsp olive oil
- 4 tsp lemon juice
- Pinch black pepper, ground and salt
- 4 tsp oregano, chopped
- 1 small habanero pepper, chopped
- ¼ cup green onions, chopped
- 1 cup red bell pepper, chopped

DIRECTIONS

1. In a bowl (medium-size), combine the green onion, ¼ cup lemon juice, bell pepper, habanero, garlic clove, oregano, black pepper, and salt.
2. In another bowl, mix the paprika, 4 tsp lemon juice, olive oil, and garlic clove.
3. Stir the mix, coat the fish with this mix; set aside for 10 minutes.
4. Add the fish to the preheated grill over a medium-high heat setting.
5. Season the fish with black pepper and salt, and cook for 5 minutes on each side.
6. Add between serving plates, top with the salsa, and serve.

NUTRITION

Calories: 201 Kcal; Protein: 23 g; Carbohydrates: 14 g; Fat: 6 g

FISH CURRY DINNER

INGREDIENTS

- 1 tbsp red curry paste
- 1½ cups chicken broth
- 1 (14-oz.) can of coconut milk
- 1 tbsp avocado oil
- ½ cup white onion, diced
- 2 garlic cloves, minced
- ½ tsp coconut sugar
- 1 tsp salt
- ½ tsp black pepper, ground
- 4 (4-oz.) halibut fillets

DIRECTIONS

1. In a skillet (you can also use a saucepan); heat the oil over the medium stove flame.
2. Add the onions, and garlic, stir the mixture, and cook while stirring for about 2–3 minutes until softened.
3. Stir in the paste. Add the broth, coconut milk, coconut sugar, salt, and pepper; combine well.
4. Place the heat to low then simmer for 8-10 minutes.
5. Add the fillets; cover and cook for 8-10 minutes, until flakes easily.
6. Serve the fillets with the curried broth.

4 minutes

30 minutes

4

NUTRITION

Calories: 418 Kcal; Protein: 29 g; Carbohydrates: 13 g; Fat: 21 g

SALMON BROCCOLI BOWL

INGREDIENTS

- 3 tbsp avocado oil
- 2 garlic cloves, minced
- 1 broccoli head, separate florets
- 1 ½ lb. salmon fillets, boneless
- Pinch black pepper, ground and salt
- Juice of ½ lemon

DIRECTIONS

1. Preheat an oven to 450°F. Line a baking sheet with foil.
2. Spread the broccoli; add the salmon, oil, garlic, salt, pepper, and lemon juice, and toss gently.
3. Bake for 15 minutes.
4. Divide into serving plates and serve warm.

5 minutes

20 minutes

4

NUTRITION

Calories: 420 Kcal; Protein: 34 g; Carbohydrates: 7 g; Fat: 21 g

FENNEL BAKED COD

10 minutes

25 minutes

4

INGREDIENTS

- 3 sun-dried tomatoes, chopped
- 1 small red onion, (cut into slices)
- ½ fennel bulb, (cut into slices)
- 2 cod fillets, boneless
- 1 garlic clove, minced
- 1 tsp olive oil
- Black pepper to taste
- 4 black olives, pitted and sliced
- 2 rosemary springs
- ¼ tsp red pepper flakes

DIRECTIONS

1. Preheat an oven to 400°F. Grease a baking dish with a cooking spray.
2. Add the cod, garlic, black pepper, tomatoes, onion, fennel, olives, rosemary, and pepper flakes; mix gently.
3. Bake for 14–15 minutes.
4. Divide the fish mix between plates and serve.

NUTRITION

Calories: 350 Kcal; Protein: 20 g; Carbohydrates: 11 g; Fat: 9 g

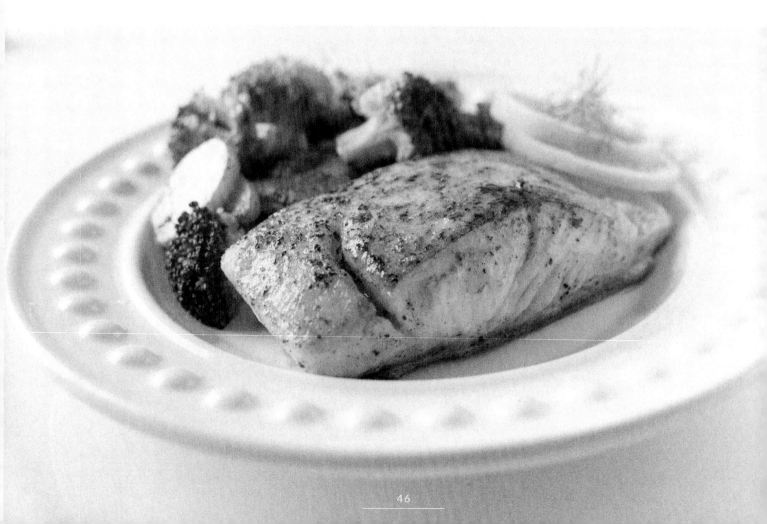

BEET HADDOCK DINNER

INGREDIENTS

- 2 tbsp olive oil
- 2 tbsp apple cider vinegar
- 1 tsp fresh thyme, chopped
- 8 beets, peeled and cut into small chunks
- 2 shallots, (cut into slices)
- 1 tsp garlic, minced
- Pinch sea salt to taste
- 4 (5-oz.) haddock fillets, patted dry

DIRECTIONS

1. Preheat an oven to 400°F. Grease a baking dish with a cooking spray.
2. In a bowl (medium size), mix the beets, shallots, garlic, and 1 tbsp olive oil.
3. Add the beet mixture to the baking dish.
4. Bake for about 25–30 minutes, or until the vegetables are caramelized.
5. Remove from the oven and stir in the cider vinegar, thyme, and sea salt.
6. In a skillet (you can also use a saucepan); heat the remaining oil over the medium stove flame.
7. Add the fish, stir the mixture and cook whilst stirring for 12–15 minutes until well cooked.
8. Flake the fish and serve with roasted beets.

10 minutes

40-45 minutes

4

NUTRITION

Calories: 500 Kcal; Protein: 50 g; Carbohydrates: 69 g; Fat: 9 g

HONEY SCALLOPS

INGREDIENTS

- 1-lb. large scallops, rinsed
- Dash black pepper, ground and salt, to taste
- 3 tbsp coconut aminos
- 2 garlic cloves, minced
- 2 tbsp avocado oil
- ¼ cup raw honey
- 1 tbsp apple cider vinegar

DIRECTIONS

1. Sprinkle the scallops with salt and pepper.
2. In a skillet (you can also use a saucepan); heat the oil over the medium stove flame.
3. Add the scallops, stir the mixture and cook while stirring for about 2–3 minutes until softened and golden.
4. Transfer to a plate, and set aside.
5. In the same skillet or pan, heat the honey, coconut aminos, garlic, and vinegar.
6. Cook for 6–7 minutes; add the scallops and coat well. Serve warm.

5 minutes

25 minutes

4

NUTRITION

Calories: 672 Kcal; Protein: 43 g; Carbohydrates: 33 g; Fat: 23 g

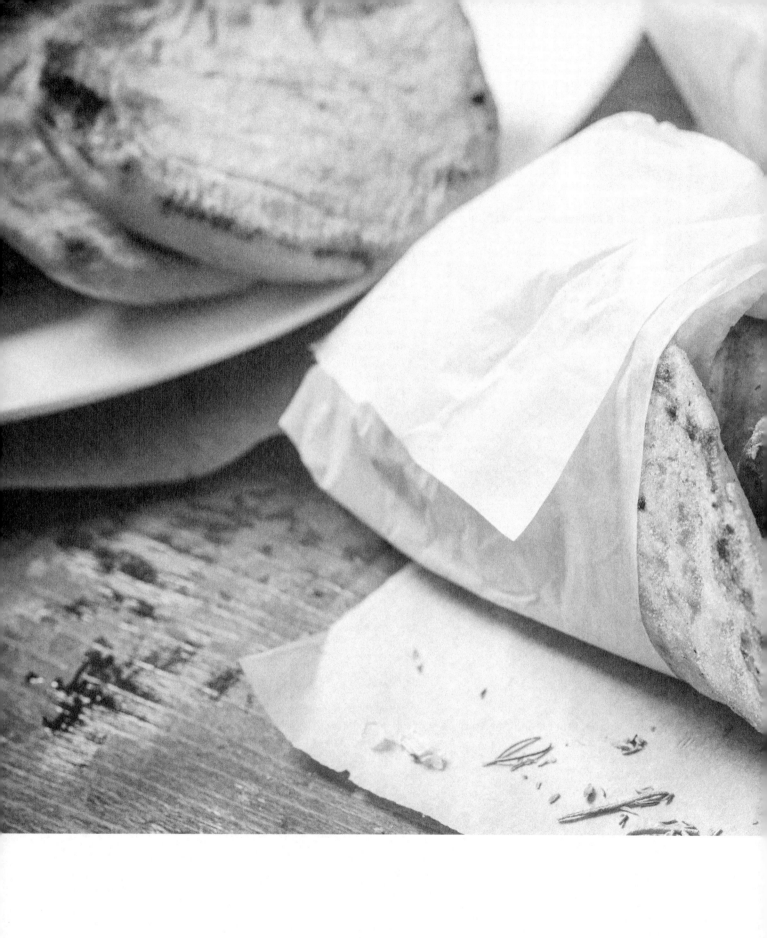

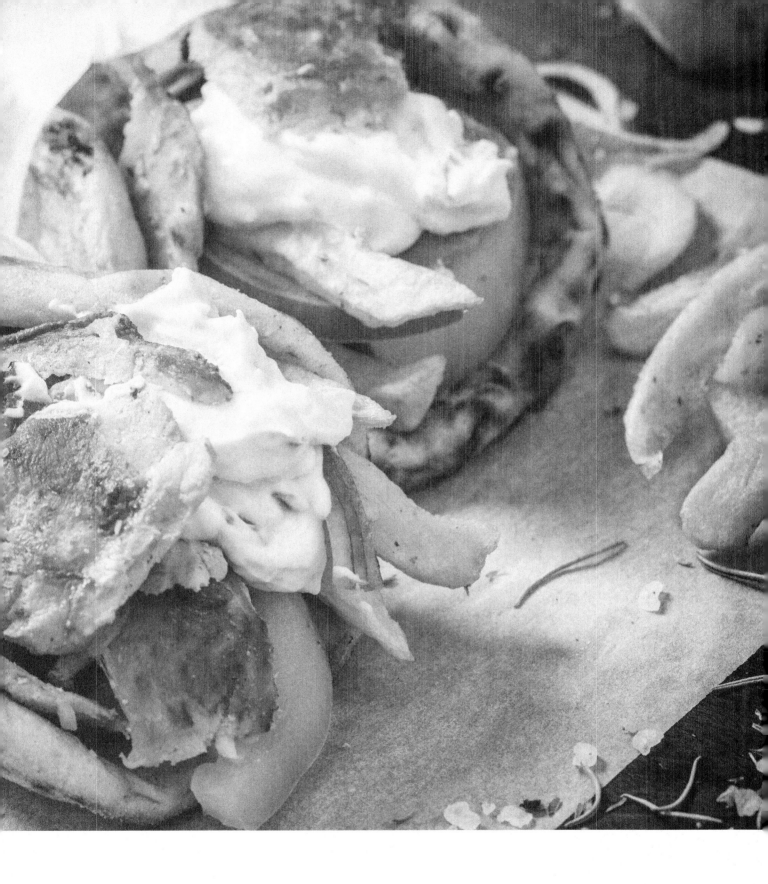

37

GROUND LAMB WITH PEAS

15 minutes

55 minutes

4

INGREDIENTS

- 1 tbsp coconut oil
- 3 red chilies, dried
- 1 (2") cinnamon stick
- 3 green cardamom pods
- ½ tsp cumin seeds
- 1 medium red onion, chopped
- 1 (¾") piece fresh ginger, minced
- 4 garlic cloves, minced
- 1½ tsp coriander, ground
- ½ tsp garam masala
- ½ tsp cumin, ground
- ½ tsp turmeric, ground
- ¼ tsp nutmeg, ground
- 2 bay leaves
- 1-lb. lean lamb, ground
- ½ cup Roma tomatoes, chopped
- 1-1½ cups of water
- 1 cup fresh green peas, shelled
- 2 tbsp plain Greek yogurt, whipped
- ¼ cup fresh cilantro, sliced
- Salt and black pepper, freshly ground

DIRECTIONS

1. In a Dutch oven, melt coconut oil on medium-high heat.
2. Add red chilies, cinnamon sticks, cardamom pods, cumin seeds, and sauté for around 30 seconds.
3. Add onion and sauté for about 3–4 minutes.
4. Add ginger, garlic cloves, spices, and sauté for around 30 seconds.
5. Add lamb and cook for approximately 5 minutes.
6. Add tomatoes and cook for 10 min.
7. Stir in water and green peas and cook, covered for 25–30 minutes.
8. Stir in yogurt, cilantro, salt, and black pepper, and cook for around 4-5 minutes.
9. Serve hot.

NUTRITION

Calories: 1200 Kcal; Protein: 80 g; Carbohydrates: 45 g; Fat: 30 g

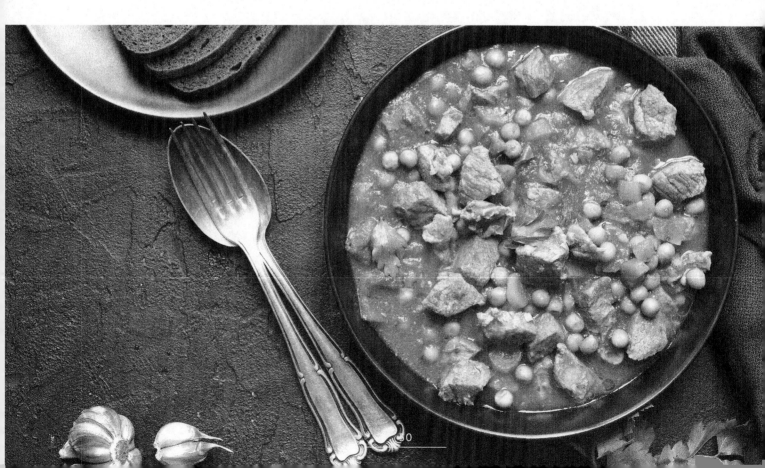

STEAK AND ONION SANDWICH

INGREDIENTS

- 4 flank steaks (around 4 oz. each)
- 1 medium red onion, sliced
- 1 tbsp lemon juice
- 1 tbsp Italian seasoning
- 1 tsp black pepper
- 1 tbsp vegetable oil
- 4 sandwich/burger buns

DIRECTIONS

1. Wrap the steak with lemon juice, Italian seasoning, and pepper to taste. Cut into four pieces. Heat the vegetable oil in a medium skillet over medium heat.
2. Cook steaks for around 3 minutes on each side until you get a medium to well-done result. Take off and transfer onto a dish with absorbing paper.
3. In the same skillet, sauté the onions until tender and transparent (around 3 minutes).
4. Cut the sandwich bun into half and place one piece of steak in each topped with the onions. Serve or wrap with paper or foil and keep in the fridge for the next day.

5 minutes

8 minutes

4

NUTRITION

Calories: 906 Kcal; Protein: 80 g; Carbohydrates: 50 g; Fat: 30 g

PESTO PORK CHOPS

INGREDIENTS

- 4 (3-oz.) pork top-loin chops, boneless, fat trimmed
- 8 tsp herb pesto
- ½ cup breadcrumbs
- 1 tbsp olive oil

DIRECTIONS

1. Preheat the oven to 450°F.
2. Line a baking sheet with foil. Set aside.
3. Rub 1 tsp of pesto evenly over both sides of each pork chop.
4. Lightly dredge each pork chop in the breadcrumbs.
5. Heat the oil in a skillet.
6. Brown the pork chops on each side for 5 minutes.
7. Place the pork chops on the baking sheet.
8. Bake for 10 minutes or until pork reaches 145°F in the center.

20 minutes

20 minutes

4

NUTRITION

Calories: 439 Kcal; Protein: 19 g; Carbohydrates: 13 g; Fat: 25 g

40

20 minutes

15 minutes

4

GRILLED STEAK WITH SALSA

INGREDIENTS

For the salsa:

- 1 cup English cucumber, chopped
- ¼ cup red bell pepper, boiled and diced
- 1 Scallion both green and white parts, chopped
- 2 tbsp fresh cilantro chopped
- Juice of 1 lime

For the steak:

- 4 (3-oz.) Beef tenderloin steaks, room temperature
- Olive oil
- Black pepper, freshly ground

DIRECTIONS

1. In a bowl, to make the salsa, combine the lime juice, cilantro, scallion, bell pepper, and cucumber. Set aside.
2. Preheat a barbecue to medium heat to cook the steaks.
3. Rub the steaks with oil and season with pepper.
4. Grill the steaks for around 5 minutes on each side for medium-rare, or until the desired doneness.
5. Serve the steaks topped with salsa.

NUTRITION

Calories: 450 Kcal; Protein: 35 g; Carbohydrates: 30 g; Fat: 12 g

---

41

10 minutes

8 hours

4

OREGANO PORK

INGREDIENTS

- 2 lb. pork roast, sliced
- 2 tbsp oregano, chopped
- ¼ cup balsamic vinegar
- 1 cup tomato paste
- 1 tbsp sweet paprika
- 1 tsp onion powder
- 2 tbsp chili powder
- 2 garlic cloves, minced
- A pinch of salt and black pepper

DIRECTIONS

1. In a slow cooker, combine the roast with the oregano, the vinegar, and the other ingredients, toss, put the lid on then cook on Low for 8 hours.
2. Divide everything between plates and serve.

NUTRITION

Calories: 1200 Kcal; Protein: 190 g; Carbohydrates: 73 g; Fat: 35 g

ZERO-FUSSING PORK MEAL

INGREDIENTS

- 1 lb. lean pork, cut into bite-sized cubes
- 2 potatoes, peeled and quartered
- 1 lb. fresh green beans
- 2 carrots, peeled and sliced thinly
- 2 celery stalks, sliced thinly
- 1 large onion, chopped
- 3 fresh tomatoes, grated
- ½ cup extra-virgin olive oil
- 1 tsp thyme, dried
- Salt and black pepper, freshly ground, to taste

DIRECTIONS

1. In a slow cooker, place all the ingredients and stir to combine.
2. Set the slow cooker on "High" and cook, covered for about 6 hours.
3. Serve hot.

20 minutes

6 hours

4

NUTRITION

Calories: 800 Kcal; Protein: 120.1 g; Carbohydrates: 91.3 g; Fat: 29.7 g

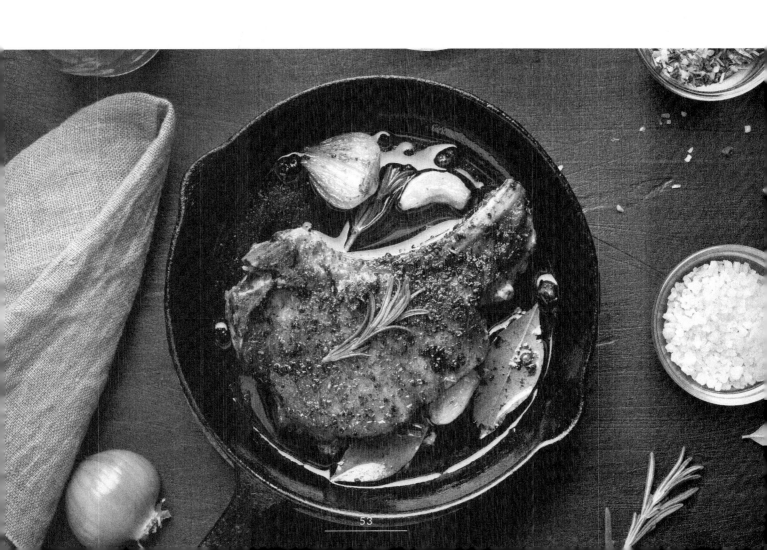

SPICY ROASTED LEG OF LAMB

30 minutes

2 hours

4

INGREDIENTS

For the lamb:

- 1 lb./450 g. leg of lamb, bone-in
- Salt and pepper
- 3 tbsp olive oil
- 5 garlic cloves, sliced
- 2 cups of water
- 4 potatoes, cubed
- 1 onion, chopped
- 1 tsp garlic powder

For the lamb spice rub:

- 15 garlic cloves, peeled
- 3 tbsp oregano
- 2 tbsp mint
- 1 tbsp paprika
- ½ cup olive oil
- ¼ cup lemon juice

DIRECTIONS

1. Allow the lamb to rest for 1 hour at room temperature.
2. While you wait, put all of the spice rub ingredients in a food processor and blend. Refrigerate the rub.
3. Make a few cuts in the lamb using a knife. Season with salt and pepper.
4. Place on a roasting pan.
5. Heat the broiler and broil for 5 minutes on each side so the whole thing is seared.
6. Place the lamb on the counter and set the oven temperature to 375°F/190°C.
7. Let the lamb cool, then fill the cuts with the garlic slices and cover with the spice rub.
8. Add 2 cups of water to the roasting pan.
9. Sprinkle the potatoes and onions with garlic powder, salt, and pepper. Arrange them around the leg of lamb.
10. Add oil to the top of the lamb and vegetables.
11. Use aluminum foil to cover the roasting pan and place it back in the oven.
12. Roast the lamb for 1 hour.
13. Discard the foil and roast for 15 more minutes.
14. Let the leg of lamb sit for 20 minutes before serving.

NUTRITION

Calories: 900 Kcal; Protein: 91 g; Carbohydrates: 150 g; Fat: 60 g

PORK AND CHESTNUTS MIX

INGREDIENTS

- 1 and ½ cups brown rice, already cooked
- 2 cups pork roast, already cooked and shredded
- 3 oz. water chestnuts, drained and sliced
- ½ cup sour cream
- A pinch of salt and white pepper

DIRECTIONS

1. In a bowl, mix the rice with the roast and the other ingredients, toss and keep in the fridge for 2 hours before serving.

NUTRITION

Calories: 926 Kcal; Protein: 61 g; Carbohydrates: 54 g; Fat: 50 g

30 minutes

0 minutes

6

STEAK WITH OLIVES AND MUSHROOMS

INGREDIENTS

- 1 lb. beef sirloin steak, boneless
- 1 large onion, sliced
- 5–6 white button mushrooms
- ½ cup green olives, coarsely chopped
- 4 tbsp extra virgin olive oil

DIRECTIONS

1. Heat-up olive oil in a heavy-bottomed skillet over medium-high heat. Brown the steaks on both sides then put them aside.
2. Gently sauté the onion in the same skillet, for 2–3 minutes, stirring occasionally . Sauté in the mushrooms and olives.
3. Return the steaks to the skillet, cover, cook for 5–6 minutes and serve.

NUTRITION

Calories: 900 Kcal; Protein: 89 g; Carbohydrates: 15 g; Fat: 58 g

20 minutes

9 minutes

6

46

GREEK PORK

10 minutes

1h 10'

8

INGREDIENTS

- 3 lb. pork roast, sliced into cubes
- ¼ cup chicken broth
- ¼ cup lemon juice
- 2 tsp oregano, dried
- 2 tsp garlic powder

DIRECTIONS

1. Put the pork in the Instant Pot.
2. In a bowl, mix all the remaining ingredients.
3. Pour the mixture over the pork.
4. Toss to coat evenly.
5. Secure the pot.
6. Choose a manual mode.
7. Cook at high pressure for 50 minutes.
8. Release the pressure naturally.

NUTRITION

Calories: 1500 Kcal; Protein: 160 g; Carbohydrates: 25 g; Fat: 80 g

47

PORK RIND SALMON CAKES

10 minutes

10 minutes

2

INGREDIENTS

- 6 oz. Alaska wild salmon, canned and drained
- 2 tbsp pork rinds, crushed
- 1 egg, lightly beaten
- 1 tbsp ghee
- ½ tbsp Dijon mustard

DIRECTIONS

1. In a medium bowl, incorporate salmon, pork rinds, egg, and 1½ tbsp of mayonnaise, and season with pink Himalayan salt and pepper.
2. With the salmon mixture, form patties the size of hockey pucks or smaller. Keep patting the patties until they keep together.
3. Position the medium skillet over medium-high heat, and melt the ghee. When the ghee sizzles, place the salmon patties in the pan. Cook for 6 minutes on both sides. Transfer the patties to a paper towel-lined plate.
4. In a small bowl, mix the remaining 1½ tbsp of mayonnaise and the mustard.
5. Serve the salmon cakes with the mayo-mustard dipping sauce.

NUTRITION

Calories: 406 Kcal; Protein: 53 g; Carbohydrates: 5 g; Fat: 21 g

ROSEMARY PORK CHOPS

48

INGREDIENTS

- 4 pork loin chops, boneless
- Salt and black pepper, to taste
- 4 garlic cloves, minced
- 1 tbsp rosemary, chopped
- 1 tbsp olive oil

DIRECTIONS

1. In a roasting pan, combine the pork chops with the rest of the ingredients, toss, and bake at 425°F for 10 minutes.
2. Reduce the heat to 350°F then cook the chops for 25 more minutes.
3. Divide the chops between plates and serve with a side salad.

NUTRITION

Calories: 435 Kcal; Protein: 47 g; Carbohydrates: 3 g; Fat: 25 g

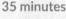

30 minutes

35 minutes

4

BEEF STEAKS WITH CREAMY BACON AND MUSHROOMS

49

INGREDIENTS

- 2 oz. bacon, chopped
- 1 cup mushrooms, sliced
- 1 garlic clove, chopped
- 1 shallot, chopped
- 1 cup heavy cream
- 1 lb. beef steaks
- 1 tsp nutmeg, ground
- ¼ cup coconut oil
- Salt and black pepper to taste
- 1 tbsp parsley, chopped

DIRECTIONS

1. Set a frying pan at medium heat, then cook the bacon for 2–3 minutes and set aside. In the same pan, warm the oil, add in the onions, garlic, and mushrooms, and cook for 4 minutes. Stir in the beef, season with salt, black pepper, and nutmeg, and sear until browned, about 2 minutes per side.
2. Preheat the oven to 360°F and insert the pan in the oven to bake for 25 minutes. Remove the beefsteaks to a bowl and cover with foil.
3. Place the pan over medium heat, pour the heavy cream over the mushroom mixture, add in the reserved bacon and cook for 5 minutes; remove from heat. Spread the bacon/mushroom sauce over beefsteaks, sprinkle with parsley and serve.

10 minutes

40 minutes

4

NUTRITION

Calories: 765 Kcal; Protein: 98 g; Carbohydrates: 5 g; Fat: 30 g

CILANTRO BEEF CURRY WITH CAULIFLOWER

6 minutes

15 minutes

3

INGREDIENTS

- 1 tbsp olive oil
- ½ lb. beef, ground
- 1 garlic clove, minced
- 1 tsp turmeric
- 1 tbsp cilantro, chopped
- 1 tbsp ginger paste
- ½ tsp gram masala
- 5 oz. whole tomatoes, canned
- 1 head cauliflower, cut into florets
- Salt and chili pepper to taste
- ¼ cup of water

DIRECTIONS

1. Warm oil in a saucepan at medium heat, and add the beef, garlic, ginger paste, and garam masala. Cook for 5 minutes while breaking any lumps.
2. Stir in the tomatoes and cauliflower, season with salt, turmeric, and chili pepper, and cook covered for 6 minutes. Add the water and bring to a boil over medium heat for 10 minutes or until the water has reduced by half. Scoop the curry into serving bowls and serve sprinkled with cilantro.

NUTRITION

Calories: 565 Kcal; Protein: 55 g; Carbohydrates: 36 g; Fat: 30 g

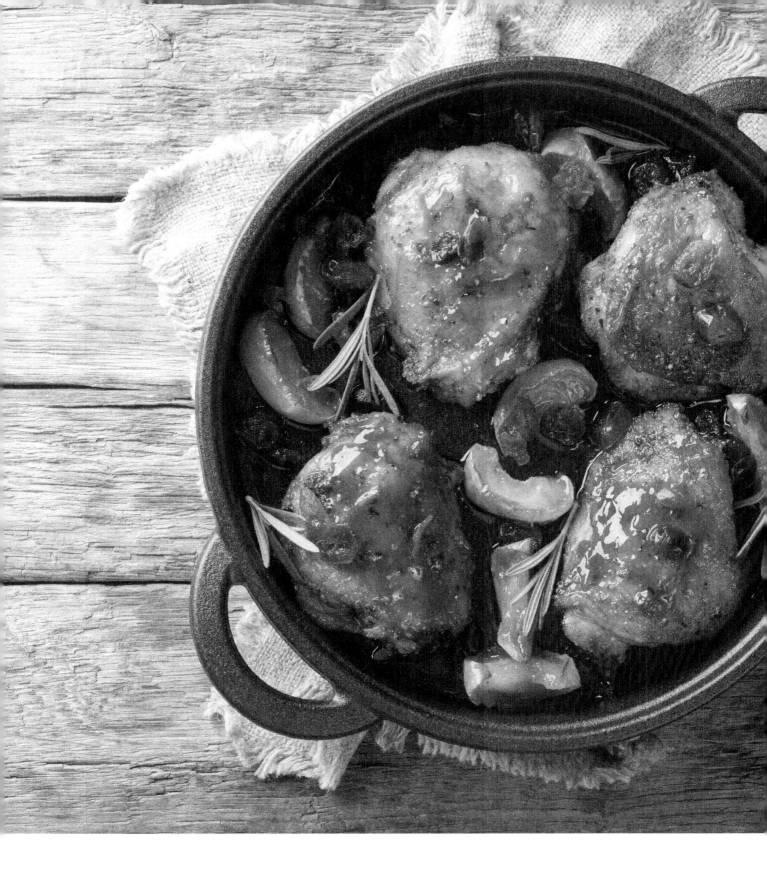

CHAPTER 5
POULTRY RECIPES

ROSEMARY CHICKEN

10 minutes

10 minutes

2

INGREDIENTS

- 2 zucchinis
- 1 carrot
- 1 tsp rosemary, dried
- 4 chicken breasts
- ½ bell pepper
- ½ red onion
- 8 garlic cloves
- 1 tbsp Olive oil
- ¼ tbsp pepper, ground

DIRECTIONS

1. Prepare the oven and preheat it to 375°F (or 200°C).
2. Slice both zucchini and carrots and add bell pepper, onion, and garlic, and put everything in a 13" x 9" pan, adding oil.
3. Spread the pepper over everything and roast for about 10 minutes.
4. Meanwhile, lift the chicken skin and spread black pepper and rosemary on the flesh.
5. Remove the vegetable pan from the oven and add the chicken, returning it to the oven for about 30 more minutes. Serve and enjoy!

NUTRITION

Calories: 597 Kcal; Protein: 67 g; Carbohydrates: 30 g; Fat: 21 g

SMOKEY TURKEY CHILI

5 minutes

45 minutes

8

INGREDIENTS

- 12 oz. lean ground turkey
- ½ red onion, chopped
- 2 garlic cloves, crushed and chopped
- ½ tsp paprika, smoked
- ½ tsp chili powder
- ½ tsp thyme, dried
- ¼ cup beef stock, reduced-sodium
- ½ cup of water
- 1 ½ cups baby spinach leaves, washed
- 3 wheat tortillas

DIRECTIONS

1. Brown the ground beef in a dry skillet over medium-high heat.
2. Add in the red onion and garlic.
3. Sauté the onion until it goes clear.
4. Transfer the contents of the skillet to the slow cooker.
5. Add the remaining ingredients and simmer on low for 30–45 minutes.
6. Stir through the spinach for the last few minutes to wilt.
7. Slice tortillas and gently toast under the broiler until slightly crispy.
8. Serve on top of the turkey chili.

NUTRITION

Calories: 900 Kcal; Protein: 73 g; Carbohydrates: 65 g; Fat: 38 g

AVOCADO-ORANGE GRILLED CHICKEN

INGREDIENTS

- ¼ cup fresh lime juice
- ¼ cup red onion, minced
- 1 avocado
- 1 cup low-fat yogurt
- 1 small red onion, sliced thinly
- 1 tbsp honey
- 2 oranges, peeled and cut
- 2 tbsp cilantro, chopped
- 4 pieces of 4-6 oz. chicken breasts, boneless, skinless
- Pepper and salt, to taste

DIRECTIONS

1. In a large bowl, mix honey, cilantro, minced red onion, and yogurt.
2. Submerge chicken into the mixture and marinate for at least 30 minutes.
3. Grease grate and preheat grill to medium-high fire.
4. Remove chicken from marinade and season with pepper and salt.
5. Grill for around 6 minutes per side or until chicken is cooked and juices run clear.
6. Meanwhile, peel the avocado and discard the seed—chop avocados and place them in a bowl. Quickly add lime juice and toss avocado to coat well with liquid.
7. Add cilantro, thinly sliced onions, and oranges into the bowl of avocado, and mix well.
8. Serve grilled chicken and avocado dressing on the side.

20 minutes

60 minutes

4

NUTRITION

Calories: 697 Kcal; Protein: 46 g; Carbohydrates: 89 g; Fats: 25 g

HERBS and LEMONY ROASTED CHICKEN

INGREDIENTS

- ½ tsp black pepper, ground
- ½ tsp mustard powder
- ½ tsp salt
- 1 3-lb whole chicken
- 1 tsp garlic powder
- 2 lemons
- 2 tbsp olive oil
- 2 tsp Italian seasoning

DIRECTIONS

1. In a small bowl, mix well black pepper, garlic powder, mustard powder, and salt.
2. Rinse chicken well and slice off giblets.
3. In a greased 9 x 13 baking dish, place chicken and add 1 ½ tsp of seasoning made earlier inside the chicken and rub the remaining seasoning around the chicken.
4. In a small bowl, blend olive oil and juice from 2 lemons. Drizzle over chicken.
5. Bake chicken in a preheated 350°F oven until juices run clear, around 1 ½ hours. Occasionally, baste the chicken with its juices.

15 minutes

1h 30'

8

NUTRITION

Calories: 2000 Kcal; Protein: 200 g; Carbohydrates: 21 g; Fats: 160 g

55

15 minutes

6-10 minutes

3-4

GROUND CHICKEN AND PEAS CURRY

INGREDIENTS

- 3 tbsp essential olive oil
- 2 bay leaves
- Onion paste (2 onions)
- ½ tbsp garlic paste
- ½ tbsp ginger paste
- 2 tomatoes, chopped finely
- 1 tbsp cumin, ground
- 1 tbsp coriander, ground
- 1 tsp turmeric, ground
- 1 tsp red chili powder
- Salt, to taste
- 1-lb. lean chicken, ground
- 2 cups peas, frozen
- 1 ½ cups of water
- 1–2 tsp garam masala powder

DIRECTIONS

1. In a deep skillet, heat-up oil on moderate heat.
2. Add bay leaves and sauté for half a minute.
3. Add onion paste and sauté for approximately 3–4 minutes.
4. Add garlic and ginger paste and sauté for around 1–1½ minutes.
5. Add tomatoes and spices and cook, occasionally stirring, for about 3–4 minutes.
6. Stir in chicken then cook for about 4–5 minutes.
7. Stir in peas and water and bring to a boil on high heat.
8. Turn the heat to low then simmer for about 5-8 minutes or till the desired doneness.
9. Stir in garam masala and remove from heat.
10. Serve hot.

NUTRITION

Calories: 1004 Kcal; Protein: 101 g; Carbohydrates: 63 g; Fat: 57 g

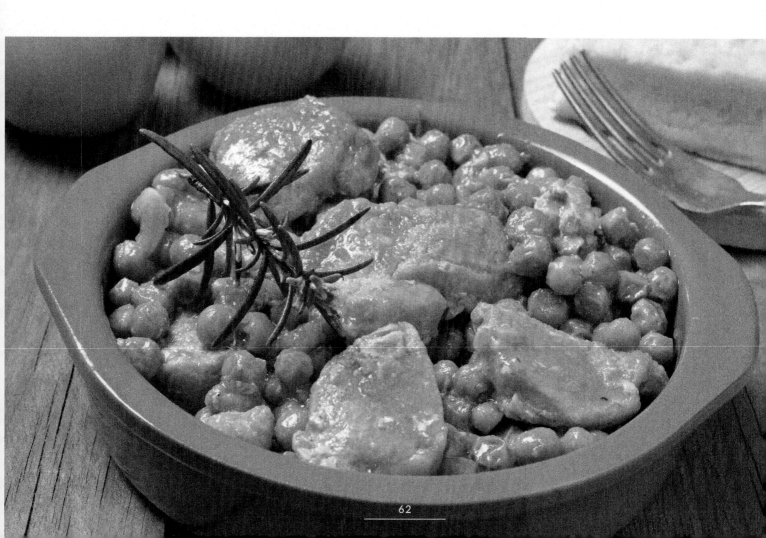

CHICKEN MEATBALLS CURRY

INGREDIENTS

For Meatballs:

- 1-lb. lean chicken, ground
- 1 tbsp onion paste
- 1 tsp fresh ginger paste
- 1 tsp garlic paste
- 1 green chili, chopped finely
- 1 tbsp fresh cilantro leaf, chopped
- 1 tsp coriander, ground
- ½ tsp cumin seeds
- ½ tsp red chili powder
- ½ tsp turmeric, ground
- Salt, to taste

For Curry:

- 3 tbsp extra-virgin olive oil
- ½ tsp cumin seeds
- 1 (1") cinnamon stick
- 3 whole cloves
- 3 whole green cardamoms
- 1 whole black cardamom
- 2 onions, chopped
- 1 tsp fresh ginger, minced
- 1 tsp garlic, minced
- 4 whole tomatoes, chopped finely
- 2 tsp coriander, ground
- 1 tsp garam masala powder
- ½ tsp nutmeg, ground
- ½ tsp red chili powder
- ½ tsp turmeric, ground
- Salt, to taste
- 1 cup of water
- Fresh cilantro, chopped, for garnishing

DIRECTIONS

1. Using a substantial bowl, add all ingredients and mix till well combined.
2. Make small equal-sized meatballs from the mixture.
3. In a big deep skillet, heat oil on medium heat
4. Add meatballs and fry for approximately 3–5 minutes or till browned on all sides.
5. Transfer the meatballs to a bowl.
6. In the same skillet, add cumin seeds, cinnamon sticks, cloves, green cardamom, and black cardamom, and sauté for approximately 1 minute.
7. Add onions and sauté for around 4–5 minutes.
8. Add ginger and garlic paste, then sauté for approximately 1 minute.
9. Add tomato and spices and cook, crushing with the back of the spoon for approximately 2–3 minutes.
10. Add water and meatballs and bring to the boil.
11. Reduce heat to low.
12. Simmer for approximately 10 minutes.
13. Serve hot with all the garnishing of cilantro.

20 minutes

25 minutes

3-4

NUTRITION

Calories: 745 Kcal; Protein: 84 g; Carbohydrates: 27 g; Fat: 50 g

PERSIAN CHICKEN

10 minutes

20 minutes

5

INGREDIENTS

- ½ sweet onion, chopped
- ¼ cup lemon juice
- 1 tbsp oregano, dried
- 1 tsp garlic, minced
- 1 tsp sweet paprika
- ½ tsp cumin, ground
- ½ cup olive oil
- 5 chicken thighs, boneless, skinless

DIRECTIONS

1. Put the cumin, paprika, garlic, oregano, lemon juice, and onion in a food processor and pulse to mix the ingredients.
2. Keep the motor running and add the olive oil until the mixture is even.
3. Put the chicken thighs in a large sealable freezer container and pour the sauce into the bag.
4. Seal the container and place it in the fridge, turning the bag 2 times for 2 hours.
5. Remove the thighs from the marinade and discard the extra marinade.
6. Preheat the barbecue to medium.
7. Grill the chicken for about 20 minutes, turning once, until it reaches 165°F.

NUTRITION

Calories: 900 Kcal; Protein: 97 g; Carbohydrates: 54 g; Fat: 43 g

CREAMY CHICKEN WITH CIDER

5 minutes

25 minutes

8

INGREDIENTS

- 4 chicken breasts, bone-in
- 2 tbsp butter, lightly salted
- ¾ cup apple cider vinegar
- ⅔ cup creamy unsweetened coconut milk or cream
- 1 tbsp Kosher pepper

DIRECTIONS

1. Melt the butter in a skillet over medium heat.
2. Season the chicken with the pepper and add to the skillet. Cook over low heat for approx. 20 minutes.
3. Remove the chicken from the heat then set it aside in a dish.
4. In the same skillet, add the cider and bring to a boil until most of it has evaporated.
5. Add the coconut cream and let cook for 1 minute until slightly thickened.
6. Pour the cider cream over the cooked chicken and serve.

NUTRITION

Calories: 535 Kcal; Protein: 60 g; Carbohydrate: 10 g; Fat: 21 g

HERBED CHICKEN

INGREDIENTS

- 12 oz. chicken breast, boneless, skinless, cut into 8 strips
- 1 egg white
- 2 tbsp water, divided
- ½ cup breadcrumbs
- ¼ cup unsalted butter, divided
- Juice of 1 lemon
- Zest of 1 lemon
- 1 tbsp fresh basil, chopped
- 1 tsp fresh thyme, chopped
- Lemon slices, for garnish

DIRECTIONS

1. Put the chicken strips between 2 sheets of plastic wrap and pound each flat with a rolling pin.
2. In a bowl, put together the egg and 1 tbsp water.
3. Put the breadcrumbs in another bowl.
4. Dip the chicken strips, one at a time, in the egg, then the breadcrumbs, and set the breaded strips aside on a plate.
5. In a large fry pan over medium heat, melt 2 tbsp of the butter.
6. Cook the breaded strips for 3 minutes, turning once, or until they are golden and cooked through. Transfer the chicken to a plate.
7. Add the lemon zest, lemon juice, basil, thyme, and remaining 1 tbsp of water to the skillet and stir until the mixture simmers.
8. Remove the sauce from the heat then mix in the remaining 2 tbsp butter
9. Serve the chicken with the lemon sauce drizzled over the top and garnish with lemon slices.

20 minutes

15 minutes

4

NUTRITION

Calories: 1083 Kcal; Protein: 94 g; Carbohydrates: 54 g; Fat: 56 g

LIME CHICKEN WITH BLACK BEANS

INGREDIENTS

- 8 chicken thighs, boneless and skinless
- 3 tbsp lime juice
- 1 cup of black beans
- 1 cup tomatoes, canned
- 4 tsp garlic powder

DIRECTIONS

1. Marinate the chicken in a mixture of lime juice and garlic powder.
2. Add the chicken to the Instant Pot.
3. Place the tomatoes on top of the chicken.
4. Seal the pot.
5. Set it to manual.
6. Cook at high pressure for 10 minutes.
7. Release the pressure naturally.
8. Stir in the black beans.
9. Press sauté to simmer until black beans are cooked.

15 minutes

30 minutes

8

NUTRITION

Calories: 1458 Kcal; Protein: 162 g; Carbohydrates: 49 g; Fat: 56 g

BALSAMIC CHICKEN

10 minutes

30 minutes

4

INGREDIENTS

- 3 chicken breasts
- ¼ cup olive oil
- ¼ cup balsamic vinegar
- 1 garlic clove

DIRECTIONS

1. In a bowl, add all ingredients.
2. Add chicken and the marinade for 3–4 hours.
3. Grill and serve with vegetables.

NUTRITION

Calories: 737 Kcal; Protein: 65 g; Carbohydrates: 5 g; Fat: 53 g

---

LEMON CHICKEN MIX

10 minutes

10 minutes

2

INGREDIENTS

- 8 oz. chicken breast, skinless, boneless
- 1 tsp Cajun seasoning
- 1 tsp balsamic vinegar
- 1 tsp olive oil
- 1 tsp lemon juice

DIRECTIONS

1. Cut the chicken breast into halves and sprinkle with Cajun seasoning.
2. Then sprinkle the poultry with olive oil and lemon juice.
3. Then sprinkle the chicken breast with balsamic vinegar.
4. Preheat the grill to 385°F.
5. Grill the chicken breast halves for 5 minutes on each side.
6. Slice Cajun chicken and place it on the serving plate.

NUTRITION

Calories: 700 Kcal; Protein: 52 g; Carbohydrates: 0.1 g; Fat: 43 g

CHICKEN SHAWARMA

INGREDIENTS

- 2 lb. chicken breast, sliced into strips
- 1 tsp paprika
- 1 tsp cumin, ground
- ¼ tsp garlic, granulated
- ½ tsp turmeric
- ¼ tsp allspice, ground

DIRECTIONS

1. Season the chicken with spices, and a little salt and pepper.
2. Pour 1 cup of chicken broth into the pot.
3. Seal the pot.
4. Choose a poultry setting.
5. Cook for 15 minutes.
6. Release the pressure naturally.

15 minutes

30 minutes

8

NUTRITION

Calories: 1184 Kcal; Protein: 214 g; Carbohydrates: 12 g; Fat: 21 g

GREEK CHICKEN BITES

INGREDIENTS

- 1-lb. chicken fillet
- 1 tbsp Greek seasoning
- 1 tsp sesame oil
- ½ tsp salt
- 1 tsp balsamic vinegar

DIRECTIONS

1. Cut the chicken into small tenders (fingers) and sprinkle them with Greek seasoning, salt, and balsamic vinegar. Mix up well with the help of the fingertips.
2. Then sprinkle chicken with sesame oil and shake gently.
3. Line the baking tray with parchment.
4. Place the marinated chicken fingers in the tray in one layer.
5. Bake the chicken fingers for 20 minutes at 355°F. Flip them to the other side after 10 minutes of cooking.

10 minutes

20 minutes

6

NUTRITION

Calories: 461 Kcal; Protein: 62 g; Carbohydrates: 2 g; Fat: 21 g

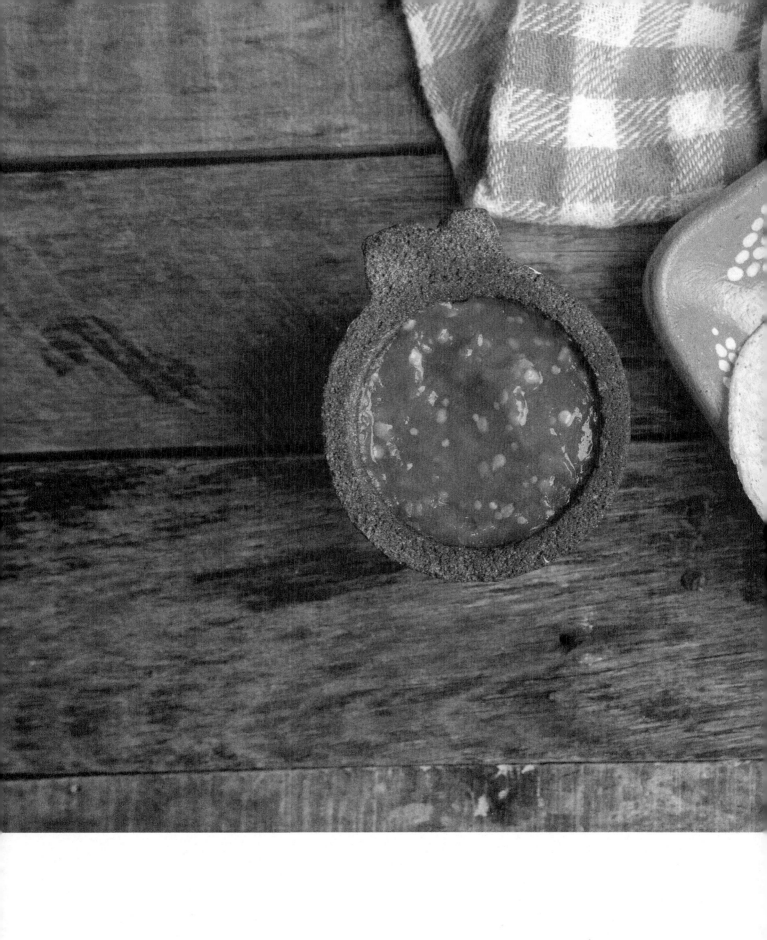

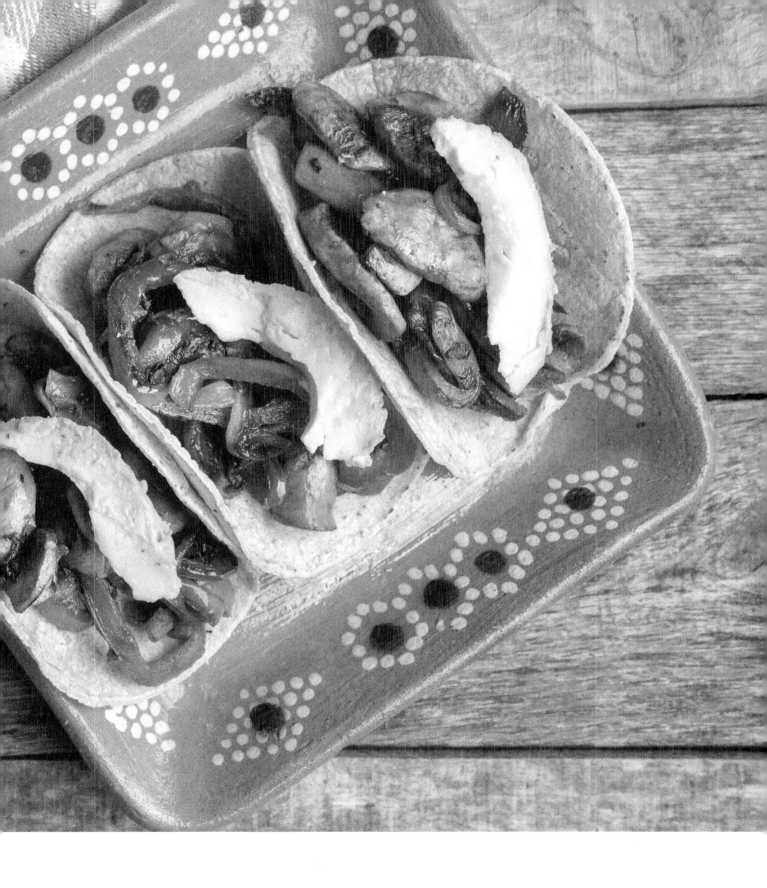

CHAPTER 6
VEGETARIAN RECIPES

65

BAKED EGGPLANT SLICES

15 minutes

15 minutes

3

INGREDIENTS

- 1 large eggplant, trimmed
- 1 tbsp butter softened
- 1 tsp minced garlic
- 1 tsp salt

DIRECTIONS

1. Cut the eggplant and sprinkle it with salt. Mix up well and leave for 10 minutes to make the vegetable "give" a bitter juice.
2. After this, dry the eggplant with a paper towel.
3. In the shallow bowl, mix up together minced garlic and softened butter.
4. Brush every eggplant slice with the garlic mixture.
5. Line the baking tray with baking paper—Preheat the oven to 355°F.
6. Place the sliced eggplants in the tray to make one layer and transfer it to the oven.
7. Bake the eggplants for 15 minutes. The cooked eggplants will be tender, but not soft!

NUTRITION

Calories: 163 Kcal; Protein: 5 g; Carbohydrates: 32 g; Fat: 5 g

---

66

PESTO AVOCADO

10 minutes

10 minutes

2

INGREDIENTS

- 1 avocado pitted, halved
- ⅓ cup Mozzarella balls, cherry size
- 1 cup fresh basil
- 1 tbsp walnut
- ¼ tsp garlic, minced
- ¾ tsp salt
- ¾ tsp black pepper, ground
- 4 tbsp olive oil
- 1 oz. Parmesan, grated
- ⅓ cup cherry tomatoes

DIRECTIONS

1. Make pesto sauce: blend salt, minced garlic, walnuts, fresh basil, ground black pepper, and olive oil.
2. When the mixture is smooth, augment grated cheese and pulse it for 3 seconds more.
3. Then scoop ½ flesh from the avocado halves.
4. In the mixing bowl, mix up together mozzarella balls and cherry tomatoes.
5. Add pesto sauce and shake it well.
6. Preheat the oven to 360°F.
7. Fill the avocado halves with the cherry tomato mixture and bake for 10 minutes.

NUTRITION

Calories: 421 Kcal; Protein: 8.2 g; Carbohydrates: 11.7 g; Fat: 43 g

Fast Cabbage Cakes

INGREDIENTS

- 1 cup cauliflower, shredded
- 1 egg, beaten
- 1 tsp salt
- 1 tsp black pepper, ground
- 2 tbsp almond flour
- 1 tsp olive oil

DIRECTIONS

1. Blend the shredded cabbage in the blender until you get cabbage rice.
2. Then, mix up cabbage rice with the egg, salt, ground black pepper, and almond flour.
3. Pour olive oil into the skillet and preheat it.
4. Then make the small cakes with the help of 2 spoons and place them in the hot oil.
5. Roast the cabbage cakes for 4 minutes from each side over medium-low heat.
6. It is suggested to use a non-stick skillet.

15 minutes

10 minutes

2

NUTRITION

Calories: 357 Kcal; Protein: 9.9 g; Carbohydrates: 9.5 g; Fat: 19.6 g

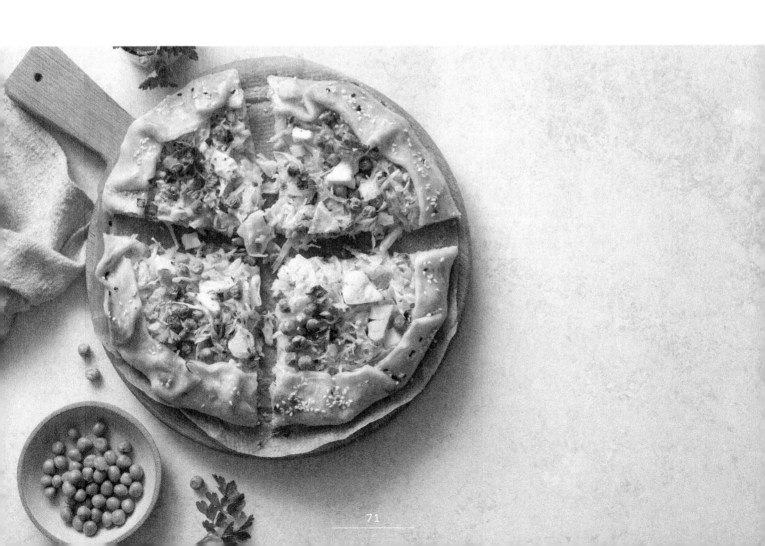

68 | VEGaN CHILI

10 minutes

20 minutes

4

INGREDIENTS

- 1 cup cremini mushrooms, chopped
- 1 zucchini, chopped
- 1 bell pepper, diced
- ⅓ cup tomatoes, crushed
- 1 oz. celery stalk, chopped
- 1 tsp chili powder
- 1 tsp salt
- ½ tsp chili flakes
- ½ cup of water
- 1 tbsp olive oil
- ½ tsp garlic, diced
- ½ tsp black pepper, ground
- 1 tsp cocoa powder
- 2 oz. Cheddar cheese, grated

DIRECTIONS

1. Pour olive oil into the pan and preheat it.
2. Add chopped mushrooms and roast them for 5 minutes. Stir them from time to time.
3. After this, add chopped zucchini and bell pepper.
4. Sprinkle the vegetables with chili powder, salt, chili flakes, diced garlic, and ground black pepper.
5. Stir the vegetables and cook them for 5 minutes more.
6. After this, add crushed tomatoes. Mix up well.
7. Bring the mixture to a boil and add water and cocoa powder.
8. Then add celery stalk.
9. Mix up the chili and close the lid.
10. Cook the chili for about 10 minutes over medium-low heat.
11. Then transfer the cooked vegan chili to the bowls and top with the grated cheese.

NUTRITION

Calories: 412 Kcal; Protein: 21,5 g; Carbohydrates: 23 g; Fat: 26 g

---

69 | MUSHROOM TacOS

10 minutes

15 minutes

6

INGREDIENTS

- 6 collard green leaves
- 2 cups mushrooms, chopped
- 1 white onion, diced
- 1 tbsp taco seasoning
- 1 tbsp coconut oil
- ½ tsp salt
- ¼ cup fresh parsley
- 1 tbsp mayonnaise

DIRECTIONS

1. Put the coconut oil in the skillet and melt it.
2. Add chopped mushrooms and diced onion. Mix up the ingredients.
3. Close the lid and cook them for 10 minutes.
4. After this, sprinkle the vegetables with Taco seasoning, and salt, and add fresh parsley.
5. Mix up the mixture and cook for 5 minutes more.
6. Then add mayonnaise and stir well.
7. Chill the mushroom mixture a little.
8. Fill the collard green leaves with the mushroom mixture and fold up them.

NUTRITION

Calories: 191 Kcal; Protein: 10 g; Carbohydrates: 20 g; Fat: 8 g

LIME SPINACH AND CHICKPEAS SALAD

INGREDIENTS

- 16 oz. chickpeas, canned, drained, and rinsed
- 2 cups baby spinach leaves
- ½ tbsp lime juice
- 2 tbsp olive oil
- 1 tsp cumin, ground
- A pinch of sea salt and black pepper
- ½ tsp chili flakes

DIRECTIONS

1. In a bowl, mix the chickpeas with the spinach and the rest of the ingredients, toss and serve cold.

10 minutes

0 minutes

4

NUTRITION

Calories: 555 Kcal; Protein: 28 g; Carbohydrates: 82 g; Fat: 18 g

CURRIED VEGGIES AND RICE

INGREDIENTS

- ¼ cup olive oil
- 1 cup long-grain white basmati rice
- 4 garlic cloves, minced
- 2½ tsp curry powder
- ½ cup shiitake mushrooms, sliced
- 1 red bell pepper, chopped
- 1 cup edamame, frozen, shelled
- 2 cups low-sodium vegetable broth
- ⅛ tsp black pepper, freshly ground

DIRECTIONS

1. Heat the olive oil in a large saucepan over medium temperature.
2. Add the rice, garlic, curry powder, mushrooms, bell pepper, and edamame; cook, stirring, for 2 minutes.
3. Add the broth and black pepper and bring to a boil.
4. Reduce the heat to low, partially cover the pot, and simmer for 15 to 18 minutes or until the rice is tender. Stir and serve.

12 minutes

18 minutes

4

NUTRITION

Calories: 399 Kcal; Protein: 16 g; Carbohydrates: 55 g; Fat: 12 g

SPICY MUSHROOM STIR-FRY

15 minutes

10 minutes

4

INGREDIENTS

- 1 cup low-sodium vegetable broth
- 2 tbsp cornstarch
- 1 tsp low-sodium soy sauce
- ½ tsp ginger, ground
- ⅛ tsp cayenne pepper
- 2 tbsp olive oil
- 2 (8-oz.) packages of button mushrooms, sliced
- 1 red bell pepper, chopped
- 1 jalapeño pepper, minced
- 3 cups of brown rice that has been cooked in unsalted water
- 2 tbsp sesame oil

DIRECTIONS

1. In a mini bowl, whisk together the broth, cornstarch, soy sauce, ginger, and cayenne pepper and set aside.
2. Warm the olive oil in a wok or heavy skillet over high heat.
3. Add the mushrooms and peppers and stir-fry for 3 to 5 minutes or until the vegetables are tender-crisp.
4. Stir the broth mixture and add it to the wok; stir-fry for 3 to 5 minutes longer or until the vegetables are tender and the sauce has thickened. Serve the stir-fry over the hot cooked brown rice and drizzle with the sesame oil.

NUTRITION

Calories: 916 Kcal; Protein: 19 g; Carbohydrates: 122 g; Fat: 38 g

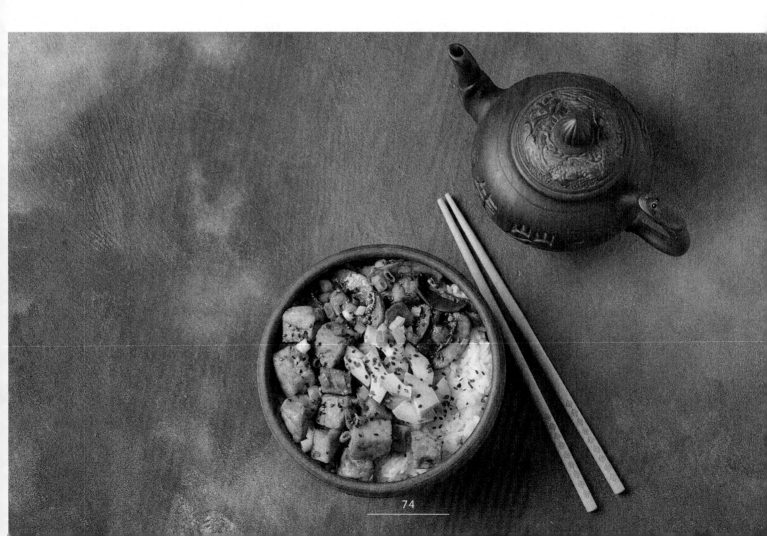

SPICY VEGGIE PANCAKES

INGREDIENTS

- 3 tbsp olive oil, divided
- 2 small onions, finely chopped
- 1 jalapeño pepper, minced
- ¾ cup carrot, grated
- ¾ cup cabbage, finely chopped
- 1½ cups quick-cooking oats
- ¾ cup brown rice, cooked
- ¾ cup of water
- ½ cup whole-wheat flour
- 1 large egg
- 1 large egg white
- 1 tsp baking soda
- ¼ tsp cayenne pepper

DIRECTIONS

1. Warm 2 tsp oil in a medium skillet over medium temperature.
2. Sauté the onion, jalapeño, carrot, and cabbage for 4 minutes.
3. While the vegetables are cooking, combine the oats, rice, water, flour, egg, egg white, cayenne pepper, and baking soda in a medium bowl until well mixed.
4. Add the cooked vegetables to the mixture and stir to combine.
5. Heat the remaining oil in a large skillet over medium heat.
6. Drop the mixture into the skillet, about ⅓ cup per pancake. Cook for 4 minutes, or until bubbles form on the pancakes' surface and the edges look cooked, then carefully flip them over.
7. Cook the other side for 3 to 5 minutes or until the pancakes are hot and firm.
8. Repeat with the remaining mixture and serve.

20 minutes

10 minutes

4

NUTRITION

Calories: 619 Kcal; Protein: 26 g; Carbohydrates: 73 g; Fat: 25 g

EGG AND VEGGIE FAJITAS

INGREDIENTS

- 3 large eggs
- 3 egg whites
- 2 tsp chili powder
- 1 tbsp butter, unsalted
- 1 onion, chopped
- 2 garlic cloves, minced
- 1 jalapeño pepper, minced
- 1 red bell pepper, chopped
- 1 cup corn, frozen, thawed, and drained
- 8 (6") corn tortillas

DIRECTIONS

1. Whisk the eggs, egg whites, and chili powder in a small bowl until well combined. Set aside.
2. In a large skillet, dissolve the butter at medium temperature.
3. Sauté the onion, garlic, jalapeño, bell pepper, and corn until the vegetables are tender, 3 to 4 minutes.
4. Put the beaten egg mixture into the skillet. Cook, occasionally stirring, until the eggs form large curds and are set, 3 to 5 minutes.
5. Meanwhile, soften the corn tortillas as directed on the package.
6. Divide the egg mixture evenly among the softened corn tortillas. Roll the tortillas up and serve.

20 minutes

10 minutes

4

NUTRITION

Calories: 891 Kcal; Protein: 43 g; Carbohydrates: 111 g; Fat: 32 g

15 minutes

15 minutes

2

TOFU AND TOMATO

INGREDIENTS

- 1 tbsp coconut oil
- A little coriander/cilantro
- 10 oz. regular firm tofu
- 2 big handfuls of baby spinach
- ½ brown onion (or red if you fancy)
- 1 handful arugula/rocket
- Black pepper, freshly ground
- 2 tomatoes
- Himalayan Sea salt
- Pinch turmeric
- A little basil
- ½ small red pepper
- A pinch of cayenne pepper

DIRECTIONS

1. Use your hands to scramble the tofu into a bowl, then chop and fry the onion quickly in a pan. Dice the peppers and do the same thing.
2. Dice the tomatoes and throw them into the pan. Toss in a pinch of turmeric and add the spinach. Add salt and grind in the pepper. Cook until the tofu is warm and cooked.
3. Throw in basil leaves, coriander, and the rocket just when the meal is about to be done. Serve with a pinch of some hot cayenne pepper.
4. You can serve it on some toasted sprouted bread with some baby spinach.

NUTRITION

Calories: 428 Kcal; Protein: 27 g; Carbohydrates: 21 g; Fat: 28 g

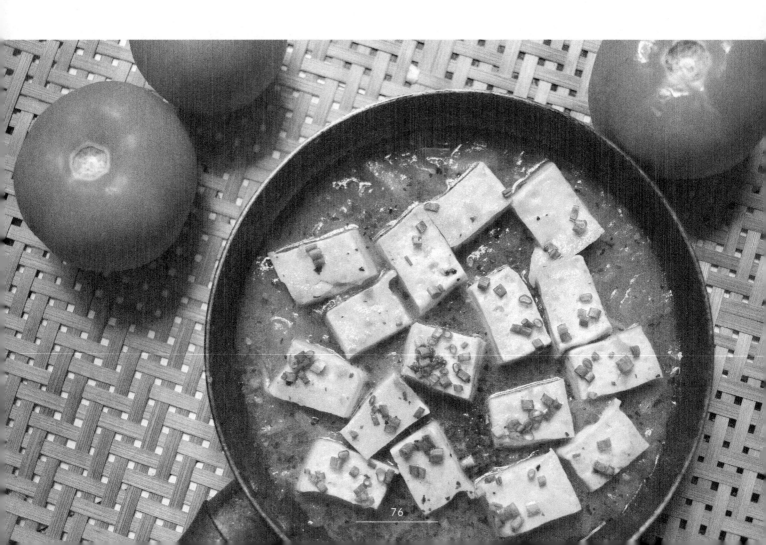

LENTIL-STUFFED POTATO CAKES

INGREDIENTS

For the cakes:

- Salt
- 1 bay leaf
- 10 medium gold potatoes
- 1 cup potato starch- add more, for dusting

For the stuffing:

- Coconut oil for pan-frying
- Salt and black pepper, freshly ground
- 1 medium onion, chopped
- 4 oz. mushrooms
- 2 tbsp olive oil
- ¾ cup green lentils, dried and cooked (preferably French lentils)

DIRECTIONS

1. Combine the 7 cups of water, potatoes, and bay leaf in a large pot and boil until the potatoes are tender. Poke with a fork to ensure they are cooked.
2. Rinse the potatoes under cold water when done; the skins will peel off easily. Now mash the potatoes until smooth and add the potato starch, stir to make the dough. Add more potato starch if the dough feels too sticky.
3. For the stuffing, add olive oil to a sauté pan and place over medium-high heat. Add in onions and cook as you stir for 5 minutes. Add in the lentils together with pepper and salt (to taste) and cook for 2 minutes. Set aside.
4. To make the cakes, scoop about 3 tbsp of the dough into your hand and press it into your palm. Add a spoonful of stuffing on top of the dough and fold it over to close it. Shape it into a round disk.
5. Now add coconut oil to a skillet and heat over medium heat. Cook the potato cakes on both sides until golden, roughly 4 minutes per side.

15 minutes

30 minutes

4

NUTRITION

Calories: 387 Kcal; Protein: 43 g; Carbohydrates: 57 g; Fat: 10 g

SESAME GINGER CAULIFLOWER RICE

10 minutes

15 minutes

4

INGREDIENTS

- 2 tbsp wheat-free tamari plus more to taste
- 4 cups of mushrooms, finely chopped
- 1 large head of cauliflower
- 2 tbsp sesame oil, toasted
- 2 tbsp grapeseed oil
- ½ tsp Celtic Sea salt, plus more to taste
- 6 green onions, finely chopped (white and green parts)
- 1 bunch cilantro, finely chopped (½ cup)
- 2 tbsp fresh ginger, minced
- 2 tsp fresh lime juice, plus more to taste
- 1 small green chili, ribbed, seeded, and minced
- 4 tsp garlic cloves, minced

DIRECTIONS

1. For the cauliflower rice, roughly cut the cauliflower into florets and get rid of the tough middle core.
2. Fit a food processor with an S blade and add the florets to pulse. Pulse for a few seconds until the florets achieve a rice-like consistency. You should have 5–6 cups of rice in the end.
3. Heat oil in a deep skillet or wok over medium-high heat and fry the ginger, green onions, chili, garlic, and mushroom seasoned with ¼ tsp of salt for 5 minutes. Once combined well and soft, add in the tamari and cauliflower rice and cook for 5 more minutes until soft.
4. Add in the remaining salt, cilantro, and lime juice and adjust the flavors as desired.
5. Serve and enjoy!

NUTRITION

Calories: 261 Kcal; Protein: 15 g; Carbohydrates: 24 g; Fat: 14 g

---

10 minutes

15 minutes

2

SPINACH WITH CHICKPEAS AND LEMON

INGREDIENTS

- 3 tbsp extra virgin olive oil
- Sea salt, to taste (i.e., Celtic Grey, Himalayan, or Redmond Real Salt)
- ½ container of grape tomatoes
- 1 large can of chickpeas, rinse well
- 1 large onion, thinly sliced
- 1 tbsp ginger, grated
- 1 large lemon, zested and freshly juiced
- 1 tsp red pepper flakes, crushed
- 4 garlic cloves, minced

DIRECTIONS

1. Pour the olive oil into a large skillet and add the onion. Cook for about 5 minutes until the onion starts to brown.
2. Add in the ginger, lemon zest, garlic, tomatoes, and red pepper flakes and cook for 3–4 minutes.
3. Toss in the chickpeas (rinsed and drained) and cook for an additional 3–4 minutes. Now add the spinach in 2 batches and once it starts to wilt, season with some sea salt and lemon juice.
4. Cook for 2 minutes.

NUTRITION

Calories: 312 Kcal; Protein: 28 g; Carbohydrates: 80 g; Fat: 9 g

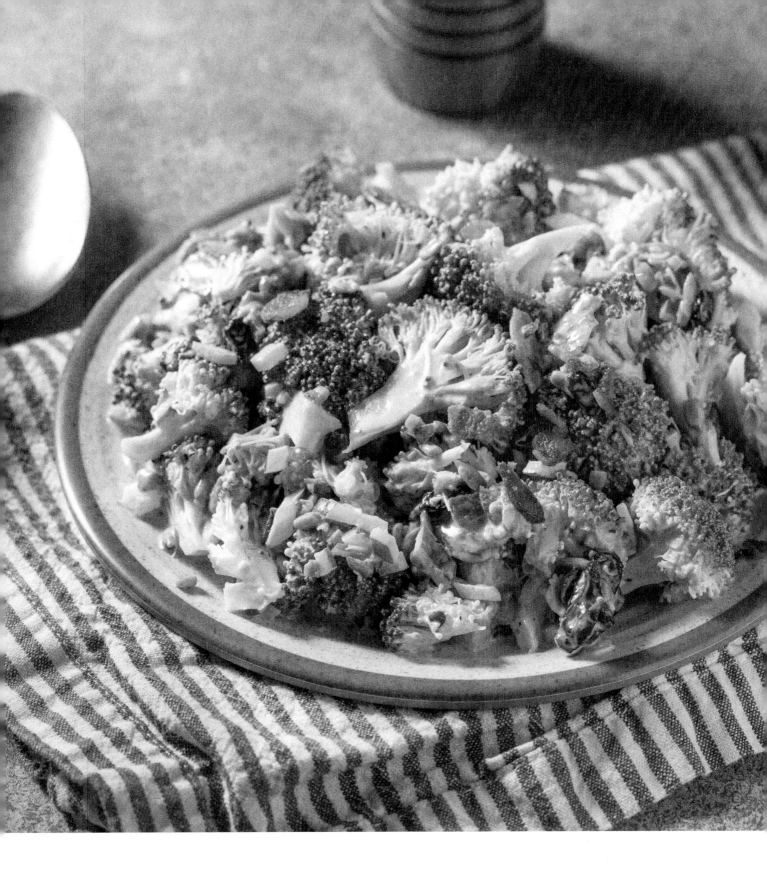

BROCCOLI SALAD

15 minutes

20 minutes

4

INGREDIENTS

For the Salad:

- Kosher salt
- 3 broccoli heads
- ½ cup Cheddar, shredded
- ¼ red onion
- ¼ cup almond, toasted
- 3 slices of bacon
- 2 tbsp fresh chives

For the dressing:

- ⅔ cup mayonnaise
- 3 tbsp apple cider
- 1 tbsp Dijon mustard
- Kosher salt
- Black paper, ground

DIRECTIONS

1. Heat 6 cups of salted water in a medium pot. Then prepare a large bowl with ice water. Mix in the broccoli florets and cook until tender. Take it out from the pan, then transfer it to the bowl with ice water. When it cools down, drain the broccoli.
2. Whisk all the dressing ingredients and season it well to your desired taste. Then mix all the salad ingredients in a separate bowl and pour the dressing. Toss it well until fully coated. Let it chill before serving.

NUTRITION

Calories: 912 Kcal; Protein: 55 g; Carbohydrates: 127 g; Fat: 21 g

---

TOMATO, CUCUMBER, AND RED ONION SALAD

20 minutes

0 minute

INGREDIENTS

- 2 large cucumbers
- 3 large tomatoes
- ⅔ cup red onion, chopped
- ⅓ cup balsamic vinegar
- ½ tbsp white sugar
- 3 tbsp extra virgin coconut oil
- Salt and pepper, to taste
- Fresh basil for garnish

DIRECTIONS

1. Combine all the ingredients and toss them well until fully coated.
2. Season it to your taste.

NUTRITION

Calories: 263 Kcal; Protein: 12 g; Carbohydrates: 30 g; Fat: 15 g

Hot Cabbage Quartet Salad

INGREDIENTS

- 3 tbsp extra-virgin olive oil
- ½ yellow onion, rinsed and finely chopped
- 8 oz. cabbage, rinsed, and shredded
- 8 oz. broccoli, rinsed, and cut into medium-sized pieces
- 8 oz. Bok choy, rinsed and chopped
- 8 oz. Brussel sprouts, rinsed and halved
- 1 tbsp celery, rinsed and finely chopped
- 1½ tsp fresh thyme leaves, rinsed and finely chopped
- 1 tsp garlic powder
- ½ tsp Himalayan pink salt, plus more as needed
- ½ tsp black pepper, freshly ground
- ¾ cup water, filtered
- 1 tbsp lemon juice, freshly squeezed

DIRECTIONS

1. Coat the interior of an electric pressure cooker with olive oil. In the pot, combine the onion, cabbage, broccoli, bok choy, brussel sprouts, celery, thyme, garlic powder, salt, and pepper. Stir well. Add the water and stir again.
2. Seal the lid into place, set Manual and High Pressure, and cook for 6 minutes.
3. When the beep sounds, quickly release the pressure by pressing Cancel and twisting the steam valve to the Venting position. Carefully remove the lid and transfer the vegetables to a serving bowl.
4. Taste and season with salt, as needed. Drizzle with the lemon juice and serve.

5 minutes

15 minutes

4

NUTRITION

Calories: 405 Kcal; Protein: 21 g; Carbohydrates: 57 g; Fat: 16 g

Tabbouleh Salad

INGREDIENTS

- 2 cups water, filtered
- 1 cup millet, rinsed
- ⅓ cup extra-virgin olive oil
- Juice of 1 lemon
- 1 large garlic clove, crushed
- 1½ tsp Himalayan pink salt, divided
- 2 large tomatoes, rinsed and finely diced
- 3 scallions, white parts only, rinsed and thinly sliced
- ½ English cucumber, rinsed and finely diced
- ¾ cup fresh mint, rinsed and finely chopped
- 1½ cup fresh parsley, rinsed and finely chopped

DIRECTIONS

1. Boil water over high heat. Add the millet and turn the heat to low. Cover the pan and cook for 15 minutes.
2. Remove the pan from the heat and mash the millet with a fork. Let cool with the lid off for 15 minutes. It should be firm but not crunchy or mushy.
3. Meanwhile, in a small bowl, whisk the olive oil, lemon juice, garlic, and ½ tsp of salt. Let sit.
4. In a large bowl, combine the tomatoes, scallions, cucumber, mint, and parsley. Add the cooled millet. Pour the dressing over and mix well. Taste and season with the remaining 1 tsp of salt, as needed.

20 minutes

15 minutes

4

NUTRITION

Calories: 360 Kcal; Protein: 8 g; Carbohydrates: 44 g; Fat: 20 g

83

10 minutes

0 minute

2

GUACAMOLE SALAD

INGREDIENTS

- 2 avocados, halved and pitted
- ½ cup red onion, diced
- ½ cup fresh cilantro, rinsed and chopped
- Juice of ½ lime
- ½ tsp onion powder
- ½ tsp cayenne, ground
- ½ tsp Himalayan pink salt
- 1 tomato, rinsed and diced

DIRECTIONS

1. Put the avocado flesh into a medium bowl. Stir in the red onion, cilantro, lime juice, onion powder, cayenne, and salt. Mash everything until smooth.
2. Add the tomato, mix well, and serve.

NUTRITION

Calories: 450 Kcal; Protein: 16 g; Carbohydrates: 27 g; Fat: 40 g

---

84

10 minutes

15 minutes

2

BUCKWHEAT SALAD

INGREDIENTS

- 1 cup raw buckwheat, rinsed
- 2 cups of water
- 2 handfuls of fresh baby spinach leaves, rinsed
- Handful of fresh basil leaves, rinsed
- 2 scallions, white parts only, rinsed and chopped
- Zest of 1 lemon
- Juice of ½ lemon
- ½ red onion, finely chopped
- Himalayan pink salt
- Black pepper, freshly ground
- ¼ cup extra-virgin olive oil
- 1 red chili, rinsed and thinly sliced
- 2 tbsp mixed sprouts, rinsed
- 1 ripe avocado, peeled, pitted, and sliced
- 1½ oz. feta cheese (optional)

DIRECTIONS

1. Mix the buckwheat and water, then bring it to a boil over high heat. Reduce the heat to simmer and cook for 15 minutes, or until soft. Remove from the heat and let cool.
2. Meanwhile, in a food processor, combine the baby spinach, basil, scallions, lemon zest, and lemon juice, and process for 30 seconds. Stir the herb mixture into the cooled buckwheat.
3. Add the red onion and season with salt and pepper. Arrange the buckwheat on a platter. Drizzle with the olive oil and scatter on the chopped chili and sprouts. Top with the sliced avocado, crumble the feta over top (if using), and serve.

NUTRITION

Calories: 685 Kcal; Fiber: 16 g; Carbohydrates: 43 g; Fat: 54 g

MIXED SPROUTS SALAD

INGREDIENTS

- 1–2 tbsp coconut oil
- Juice of 1 lemon
- Handful of fresh chives, rinsed and chopped
- Handful of fresh dill, rinsed and chopped
- Handful of fresh parsley, rinsed and chopped
- ½ tsp Himalayan pink salt
- ½ tsp black pepper, freshly ground
- 1 scallion, rinsed and chopped
- 1 cucumber, rinsed and chopped
- ½ cup mixed sprouts of choice (alfalfa, radish, broccoli, mung bean, cress, etc.), rinsed

DIRECTIONS

1. In a blender, combine the coconut oil, lemon juice, chives, dill, parsley, salt, and pepper, and blend until mainly smooth.
2. Transfer to a medium bowl. Stir in the scallion, cucumber, and sprouts to coat, and serve.

10 minutes

0 minute

2

NUTRITION

Calories: 168 Kcal; Protein: 20 g; Carbohydrates:12 g; Fat: 14 g

SWEET POTATO SALAD

INGREDIENTS

For the dressing:

- ½ cup sesame oil
- 2 tbsp coconut oil
- 2 tbsp light soy sauce
- 1 tbsp coconut sugar or raw honey
- 1 garlic clove, crushed

For the salad:

- 5 ½ oz. fresh baby spinach leaves, rinsed
- 1 red onion, rinsed and finely chopped
- 1 tomato, rinsed, seeded, and chopped
- 1 tbsp coconut oil
- 1 large, sweet potato, scrubbed, peeled, and diced

DIRECTIONS

To make the dressing:

1. In a small bowl, whisk the sesame oil, coconut oil, soy sauce, coconut sugar, and garlic until blended. Set aside.

To make the salad:

2. In a large salad bowl, gently toss together the baby spinach, red onion, and tomato. Set aside.
3. In a small skillet over medium heat, heat the coconut oil. Add the sweet potato and cook for 3–5 minutes, stirring, until golden brown. Using a slotted spoon, add the sweet potato to the salad and gently stir to combine. Pour the dressing over the salad, gently toss again to coat, and serve.

15 minutes

5 minutes

2

NUTRITION

Calories: 550 Kcal; Protein: 42 g; Carbohydrates: 20 g; Fat: 52 g

WALDORF SALAD

15' + overnight to soak

0 minute

2

INGREDIENTS

For the dressing:

- 1 ripe avocado, peeled and pitted
- 1 tsp Dijon mustard
- ½ tsp Himalayan pink salt
- Black pepper, freshly ground
- Juice of ½ lemon

For the salad:

- 2 cups chickpeas, canned, rinsed and drained, or cooked, drained, and cooled
- 1 cup sunflower seeds, soaked in filtered water overnight, drained
- 2 apples, rinsed, cored, and chopped
- ½ red onion, rinsed and diced
- 1 celery stalk, rinsed and diced
- 1–2 tsp fresh dill, chopped and rinsed

DIRECTIONS

To make the dressing:

1. In a small bowl, using a fork, mash together the avocado, mustard, salt, pepper, and lemon juice. Set aside.

To make the salad:

2. In a large bowl, stir together the chickpeas, sunflower seeds, and dressing until well combined. Stir in the apples, red onion, and celery. Top with the fresh dill and serve.

NUTRITION

Calories: 700 Kcal; Protein: 28 g; Carbohydrates: 80 g; Fat: 40 g

---

PERSIMMON SALAD

10 minutes

0 minutes

4

INGREDIENTS

- Seeds from 1 pomegranate
- 2 persimmons, cored and sliced
- 5 cups baby arugula
- 6 tbsp green onions, chopped
- 4 navel oranges, cut into segments
- ¼ cup white vinegar
- ⅓ cup olive oil
- 3 tbsp pine nuts
- 1 and ½ tsp orange zest, grated
- 2 tbsp orange juice
- 1 tbsp coconut sugar
- ½ shallot, chopped
- A pinch of cinnamon powder

DIRECTIONS

1. In a salad bowl, combine the pomegranate seeds with persimmons, arugula, green onions, and oranges, and toss. In another bowl, combine the vinegar with the oil, pine nuts, orange zest, orange juice, sugar, shallot, and cinnamon, whisk well, add to the salad, toss and serve as a side dish.

NUTRITION

Calories: 800 Kcal; Protein: 16 g; Carbohydrates: 179 g; Fat: 23 g

AVOCADO SIDE SALAD

INGREDIENTS

- 4 blood oranges, slice into segments
- 2 tbsp olive oil
- A pinch of red pepper, crushed
- 2 avocados, peeled, cut into wedges
- 1 and ½ cups baby arugula
- 1 tbsp lemon juice

DIRECTIONS

1. Mix the oranges with the oil, red pepper, avocados, arugula, almonds, and lemon juice in a bowl, and then serve.

10 minutes

0 minutes

4

NUTRITION

Calories: 848 Kcal; Protein: 12 g; Carbohydrates: 90 g; Fat: 50 g

MINTY OLIVES AND TOMATOES SALAD

INGREDIENTS

- 1 cup Kalamata olives
- 1 cup black olives
- 1 cup cherry tomatoes
- 4 tomatoes
- 1 red onion, chopped
- 2 tbsp oregano, chopped
- 1 tbsp mint, chopped
- 2 tbsp balsamic vinegar
- ¼ cup olive oil
- 2 tsp Italian herbs, dried

DIRECTIONS

1. In a salad bowl, mix the olives with the tomatoes and the rest of the ingredients, toss, and serve cold.

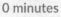

10 minutes

0 minutes

4

NUTRITION

Calories: 883 Kcal; Protein: 5 g; Carbohydrates: 55 g; Fat: 63 g

10 minutes

0 minutes

4

BEANS AND CUCUMBER SALAD

INGREDIENTS

- 15 oz. great northern beans, canned
- 2 tbsp olive oil
- ½ cup baby arugula
- 1 cup cucumber
- 1 tbsp parsley
- 2 tomatoes, cubed
- 2 tbsp balsamic vinegar

DIRECTIONS

1. Mix the beans with the cucumber and the rest of the ingredients in a large bowl, toss and serve cold.

NUTRITION

Calories: 825 Kcal; Protein: 56 g; Carbohydrates: 134 g; Fat: 9 g

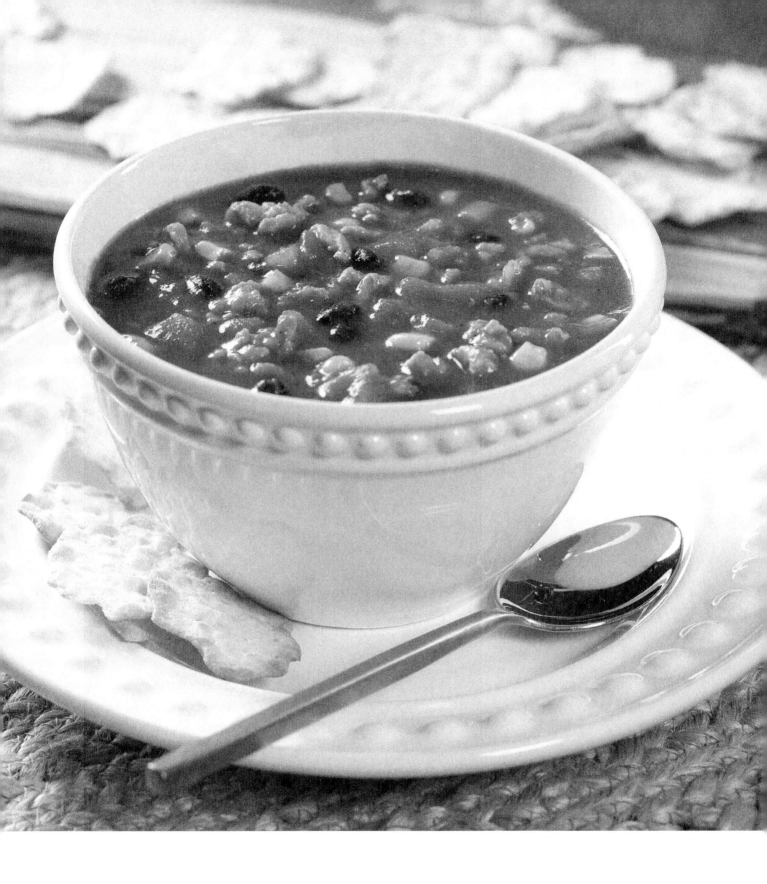

CHAPTER 8
SOUP RECIPES

CHICKEN SQUASH SOUP

15 minutes

5h 30'

3

INGREDIENTS

- ½ large butternut squash
- 1 garlic clove
- 1 ¼ quarts broth (vegetable or chicken)
- ⅛ tsp white pepper
- ½ tbsp parsley, chopped
- 2 sage leaves, minced
- 1 tbsp olive oil
- ¼ white onion, chopped
- tsp black pepper, cracked
- ½ tbsp chili pepper flakes
- ½ tsp rosemary, chopped

DIRECTIONS

1. Preheat the oven to 400°F. Grease a baking sheet. Roast the squash in a preheated oven for 30 min. Transfer it to a plate and let it cool. Sauté onion and garlic in the oil.
2. Now, scoop out the flesh from the roasted squash and add to the sautéed onion and garlic. Mash all of it well. Pour ½ quart of the broth into the slow cooker. Add the squash mixture. Cook on "low" for 4 hrs. Using a blender, make a smooth puree.
3. Transfer the puree to the slow cooker. Add in the rest of the broth and other ingredients. Cook again for 1 hr. on "high." Serve in heated soup bowls.

NUTRITION

Calories: 321 Kcal; Protein: 12 g; Carbohydrates: 54 g; Fats: 16 g

VEGGIE AND BEEF SOUP

15 minutes

4 hours

4

INGREDIENTS

- 1 carrot, chopped
- 1 celery rib, chopped
- ¾ l. sirloin, ground
- 1 cup of water
- ½ large butternut squash
- 1 garlic clove
- ½ quart beef broth
- 7 oz. tomatoes, unsalted and diced
- ½ tsp kosher salt
- 1 tbsp parsley, chopped
- ¼ tsp thyme, dried
- ¼ tsp black pepper, ground
- ½ bay leaf

DIRECTIONS

1. Sauté all the vegetables in oil. Put the vegetables to the side, then place the sirloin in the center. Sauté, using a spoon to crumble the meat. When cooked, combine with the vegetables on the sides of the pan.
2. Now, pour the rest of the ingredients into the slow cooker. Add cooked meat and vegetables. Stir well. Cook on "low" for 3 hrs. Serve in soup bowls.

NUTRITION

Calories: 268 Kcal; Protein: 9 g; Carbohydrates: 21 g; Fats: 5 g

COLLARD, SWEET POTATO, AND PEA SOUP

INGREDIENTS

- 3 ½ oz. ham steak, chopped
- ½ yellow onion, chopped
- ½ lb. sweet potatoes, sliced
- ¼ tsp red pepper, hot and crushed
- ½ cup black-eyed peas, frozen
- ½ tbsp canola oil
- 1 garlic clove, minced
- 1 ½ cup of water
- ¼ tsp salt
- 2 cups collard greens, julienned and without stems

DIRECTIONS

1. Sauté ham with garlic and onion in oil. In a slow cooker, place other ingredients except for collard greens and peas.
2. Add in the ham mixture. Cook on "low" for 3 hrs. Now, add collard green and peas and cook again for an hour on "low." Serve in soup bowls.

15 minutes

4 hours

4

NUTRITION

Calories: 463 Kcal; Protein: 26 g; Carbohydrates: 76 g; Fats: 4 g

---

BEAN SOUP

INGREDIENTS

- ½ cup pinto beans, dried
- ½ bay leaf
- 1 garlic clove
- ½ white onion
- 2 cups of water
- 2 tbsp cilantro, chopped
- 1 avocado, cubed
- ⅛ cup white onion, chopped
- ¼ cup Roma tomatoes, chopped
- 2 tbsp chipotle pepper sauce
- ¼ tsp kosher salt
- 2 tbsp cilantro, chopped
- 2 tbsp low-fat Monterrey Jack cheese, shredded

DIRECTIONS

1. Place water, salt, onion, pepper, garlic, bay leaf, and beans in the slow cooker.
2. Cook on high for 5-6 hours. Discard the Bay leaf. Serve in heated bowls.

15 minutes

5 hours

4

NUTRITION

Calories: 402 Kcal; Protein:13 g; Carbohydrates: 43 g; Fats: 27 g

BROWN RICE and CHICKEN SOUP

15 minutes

4 hours

4

INGREDIENTS

- ⅓ cups brown rice
- 1 leek, chopped
- 1 celery rib, sliced
- 1 ½ cups of water
- ½ tsp kosher salt
- ½ bay leaf
- ⅛ tsp thyme, dried
- ¼ tsp black pepper, ground
- 1 tbsp chopped parsley
- ½ quart low-sodium chicken broth
- 1 carrot, sliced
- ¾ lb. chicken thighs, skinned and boneless

DIRECTIONS

1. Boil 1 cup of water with ½ tsp of salt in a saucepan. Add the rice. Cook for 30 min. on medium flame. Brown chicken pieces in the oil. Transfer the chicken to a plate when done.
2. In the same pan, sauté the vegetables for 3 min. Now, place the chicken pieces in the slow cooker. Add water and broth. Cook on "low" for 3 hrs. Put in the rest of the ingredients, the rice last. Cook again for 10 min. on "high." After discarding Bay leaf, serve in soup bowls.

NUTRITION

Calories: 346 Kcal; Protein: 35 g; Carbohydrates: 27 g; Fats: 5 g

BUTTERNUT SQUASH SOUP

15 minutes

8 hours

6

INGREDIENTS

- 1 butternut squash, peeled, seeded, and diced
- 1 onion, chopped
- 1 sweet-tart apple (such as Braeburn), peeled, cored, and chopped
- 3 cups vegetable broth or store-bought
- 1 tsp garlic powder
- ½ tsp sage, ground
- ¼ tsp sea salt
- ¼ tsp black pepper, freshly ground
- Pinch cayenne pepper
- Pinch nutmeg
- ½ cup fat-free half-and-half

DIRECTIONS

1. In your slow cooker, combine the squash, onion, apple, broth, garlic powder, sage, salt, black pepper, cayenne, and nutmeg. Cook on low for 8 hours.
2. Using an immersion blender, counter-top blender, or food processor, purée the soup, adding the half-and-half as you do. Stir to combine and serve.

NUTRITION

Calories: 215 Kcal; Protein: 3 g; Carbohydrates: 5 5g; Fat: 0 g

CHICKPEA AND KALE SOUP

INGREDIENTS

- 1 summer squash, quartered lengthwise and sliced crosswise
- 1 zucchini, quartered lengthwise and sliced crosswise
- 2 cups chickpeas, cooked and rinsed
- 1 cup quinoa, uncooked
- 2 cans tomatoes, diced: with their juice
- 5 cups vegetable broth, poultry broth, or store-bought
- 1 tsp garlic powder
- 1 tsp onion powder
- 1 tsp thyme, dried
- ½ tsp sea salt
- 2 cups kale leaves, chopped

DIRECTIONS

1. In your slow cooker, combine the summer squash, zucchini, chickpeas, quinoa, tomatoes (with their juice), broth, garlic powder, onion powder, thyme, and salt.
2. Cover and cook on low for 8 hours. Stir in the kale.
3. Cover and cook on low for 1 more hour.

15 minutes

9 hours

6

NUTRITION

Calories: 350 Kcal; Protein: 19 g; Carbohydrates: 54 g; Fat: 3 g

CUCUMBER SOUP

INGREDIENTS

- 2 medium cucumbers
- ⅓ cup sweet white onion
- 1 green onion
- ¼ cup fresh mint
- 2 tbsp fresh dill
- 2 tbsp lemon juice
- ⅔ cup water
- ½ cup half and half cream
- ⅓ cup sour cream
- ½ tsp pepper
- Fresh dill sprigs, for garnish

DIRECTIONS

1. Place all the ingredients into a food processor and toss.
2. Puree the mixture and refrigerate for 2 hours. Garnish with dill sprigs. Enjoy fresh.

10 minutes

0 minute

4

NUTRITION

Calories: 167 Kcal; Protein: 5 g; Carbohydrates: 25 g; Fat: 6 g

SQUASH AND TURMERIC SOUP

10 minutes

30 minutes

4

INGREDIENTS

- 4 cups low-sodium vegetable broth
- 2 medium zucchini squash
- 2 medium yellow crookneck squash
- 1 small onion
- ½ cup green peas, frozen
- 2 tbsp olive oil
- ½ cup plain non-fat Greek yogurt
- 2 tsp turmeric

DIRECTIONS

1. Warm the broth in a saucepan on medium heat. Toss in onion, squash, and zucchini. Let it simmer for approximately 25 minutes then add oil and green peas.
2. Cook for another 5 minutes then allow it to cool. Puree the soup using a handheld blender then add Greek yogurt and turmeric. Refrigerate it overnight and serve fresh.

NUTRITION

Calories: 121 Kcal; Protein: 4 g; Carbohydrates: 16 g; Fat: 10 g

---

LEEK, POTATO, AND CARROT SOUP

15 minutes

25 minutes

4

INGREDIENTS

- 1 leek
- ¾ cup potatoes, diced and boiled
- ¾ cup carrots, diced and boiled
- 1 garlic clove
- 1 tbsp oil
- Pepper, crushed, to taste
- 3 cups low-sodium chicken stock
- Parsley, chopped for garnish
- 1 bay leaf
- ¼ tsp cumin, ground

DIRECTIONS

1. Trim off and take away a portion of the coarse non- useful portions of the leek, at that factor reduce daintily and flush altogether in water. Channel properly. Warm the oil in an extensively based pot. Include the leek and garlic, and sear over low warmth for 2-3 minutes, till soft.
2. Include the inventory, bay leaf, cumin, and pepper. Heat the mixture, and mix constantly. Include the bubbled potatoes and carrots and stew for 10-15 minutes. Modify the flavoring,remove the bay leaf, and serve sprinkled generously with slashed parsley.
3. To make a pureed soup, put the soup in a blender or nourishment processor till smooth. Come again to the pan. Include ½ cup of milk. Bring to bubble and stew for 2–3minutes.

NUTRITION

Calories: 391 Kcal; Protein: 30 g; Carbohydrates: 36 g; Fat: 21 g

KALE CHICKEN SOUP

INGREDIENTS

- 1 tbsp olive oil
- 3 cups kale, chopped
- 1 cup carrot, minced
- 2 cloves garlic, minced
- 8 cups chicken broth, low sodium
- sea salt and black pepper to taste
- ¾ cup patina paste, uncooked
- 2 cups chicken, cooked and shredded
- 3 tbsp parmesan cheese, grated

DIRECTIONS

1. Start by putting a stockpot over medium heat and heat your oil. Add in your garlic, cooking for half a minute. Stir frequently and add in the kale and carrots. Cook for an additional five minutes, and make sure to stir so it doesn't burn.
2. Add in salt, pepper, and broth, turning the heat to high. Boil before adding in your pasta.
3. Set the heat to medium then cook for extra 10 minutes. Your pasta should be cooked all the way through, but make sure to stir occasionally so it doesn't stick to the bottom. Add in the chicken and cook for 2 minutes.
4. Ladle the soup and serve topped with cheese.

12 minutes

18 minutes

6

NUTRITION

Calories: 761 Kcal; Protein: 95 g; Carbohydrates: 30 g; Fat: 8 g

ROASTED ROOT VEGETABLE SOUP

INGREDIENTS

- 2 parsnips, peeled and sliced
- 2 carrots, peeled and sliced
- 2 sweet potatoes, peeled and sliced
- 1 tsp fresh rosemary, chopped
- 1 tsp fresh thyme, chopped
- 1 tsp sea salt
- ½ tsp black pepper, freshly ground
- 2 tbsp extra-virgin olive oil
- 4 cups low-sodium vegetable soup
- ½ cup Parmesan cheese, grated, for garnish (optional)

DIRECTIONS

1. Preheat the oven to 400°F (205°C). Line a baking sheet with aluminum foil.
2. Combine the parsnips, carrots, and sweet potatoes in a large bowl, then sprinkle with rosemary, thyme, salt, and pepper, and drizzle with olive oil. Toss to coat the vegetables well.
3. Arrange the vegetables on the baking sheet, then roast in the preheated oven for 30 minutes or until lightly browned and soft. Flip the vegetables halfway through the roasting.
4. Pour the roasted vegetables with vegetable broth in a food processor, then pulse until creamy and smooth.
5. Pour the puréed vegetables into a saucepan, then warm over low heat until heated through.
6. Spoon the soup in a large serving bowl, then scatter with Parmesan cheese. Serve immediately.
7. Tip: If you don't have vegetable soup, just use the same amount of water to replace it.

10 minutes

35 minutes

6

NUTRITION

Calories: 260 Kcal; Protein: 12 g; Carbohydrates: 57 g; Fat: 9 g

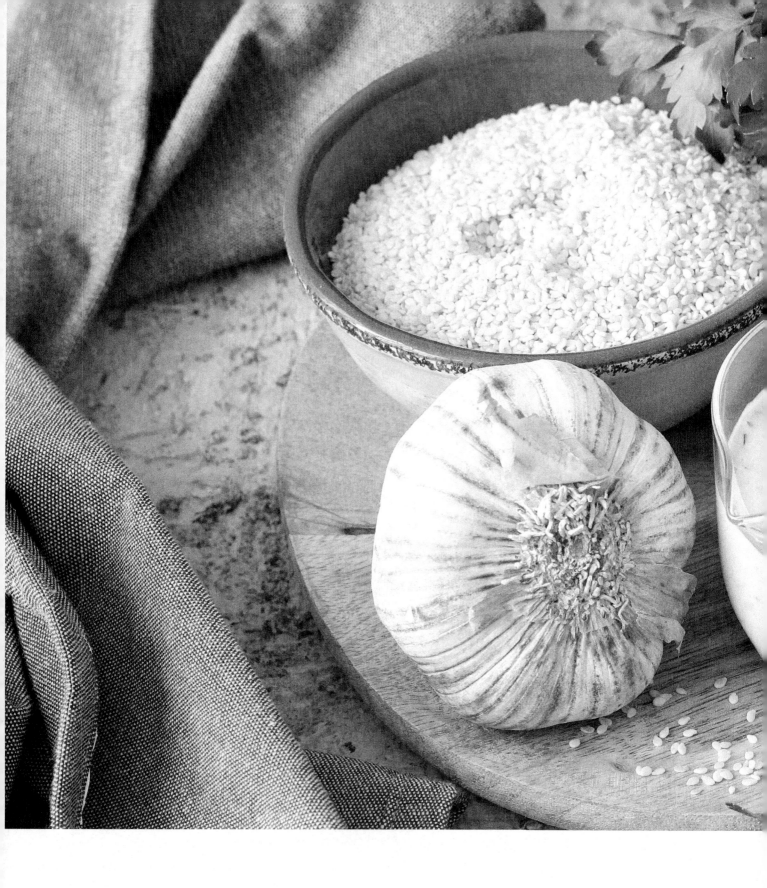

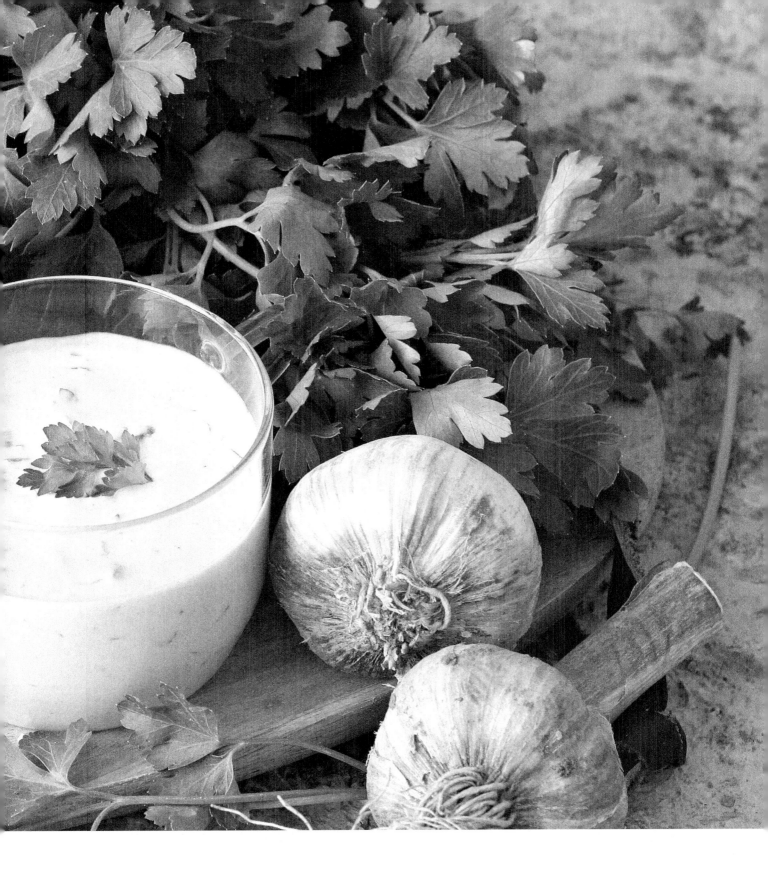

CHAPTER 9
SAUCES, CONDIMENTS, AND DRESSINGS

BLUE CHEESE DRESSING

10 minutes

0 minutes

24

INGREDIENTS

- 1 cup blue cheese, crumbled
- 1 cup sour cream
- 1 cup mayonnaise
- 2–4 drops of liquid stevia
- 2 tsp fresh lemon juice
- 2 tsp Worcestershire sauce
- 1 tsp hot pepper sauce
- 2 tbsp fresh parsley, chopped
- Salt and black pepper, ground, as required

DIRECTIONS

1. Put all the ingredients together in a large bowl and beat until well combined.
2. Refrigerate to chill before serving.

NUTRITION

Calories: 2350 Kcal; Protein: 32 g; Carbohydrate: 18 g; Fat: 190 g

---

CURRY HONEY VINAIGRETTE

10 minutes

0 minutes

¾ cup/180 ml

INGREDIENTS

- 2 tsp honey
- ¼ cup (60 ml) lime juice
- 2 tsp curry powder, plus more as needed
- ¼ tsp cayenne pepper
- ½ tsp black pepper, freshly ground
- ½ cup (120 ml) organic canola oil
- Kosher salt

DIRECTIONS

1. In a small bowl, add the honey, lime juice, curry powder, cayenne and black pepper. Whisk them together until smooth. Then whisk in the canola oil slowly until combined. Use salt to season. Taste, adding more salt or spice if desired.
2. Place in an airtight glass container, and store in the refrigerator for up to 1 week. Just before serving, whisk again to re-emulsify.

NUTRITION

Calories: 237 Kcal; Protein: 10 g; Carbohydrates: 40 g; Fat: 9 g

GARLIC PARSLEY VINAIGRETTE WITH RED WINE VINEGAR

INGREDIENTS

- 1 garlic clove, minced
- ½ cup fresh parsley, lightly packed, finely chopped
- 3 tbsp red wine vinegar
- ⅓ cup extra-virgin olive oil
- ¼ tsp salt, plus additional as needed

DIRECTIONS

1. Add the garlic, parsley, red wine vinegar, olive oil, and salt to a small jar, and combine them. Seal the jar and shake until mixed.
2. Taste the vinaigrette and adjust the seasoning as necessary.
3. Keep in the refrigerator.

NUTRITION

Calories: 261 Kcal; Protein: 3 g; Carbohydrates: 7 g; Fat: 19 g

5 minutes

0 minutes

about ½ cup

GARLIC TAHINI SAUCE WITH LEMON

INGREDIENTS

- ½ cup tahini
- 1 garlic clove, minced
- juice of 1 lemon
- zest of 1 lemon
- ½ tsp salt, plus additional as needed
- ½ cup warm water, plus additional as needed

DIRECTIONS

1. Add the tahini and garlic to a small bowl, and stir them together.
2. Stir in the lemon juice, lemon zest, and salt. Mix well.
3. Add ½ cup of warm water, and whisk until well mixed and creamy. If the sauce is too thick add more water.
4. Taste the sauce and adjust the seasoning as necessary.
5. Store in a sealed container and place in the refrigerator.

NUTRITION

Calories: 180 Kcal; Protein: 5 g; Carbohydrates: 7 g; Fat: 16 g

10 minutes

0 minutes

1 cup

EGG WHITES -GARLIC SAUCE

10 minutes

0 minutes

2 cups

INGREDIENTS

- 1 (12-oz.) organic egg whites, cooked
- 2 garlic cloves, crushed
- ½ cup fresh basil, chopped
- 1 tbsp fresh lemon juice
- ½ cup coconut oil
- 1 tsp salt
- ¼ tsp black pepper, ground

DIRECTIONS

1. Combine the egg whites, garlic, basil, lemon juice, coconut oil, salt, and pepper in a blender.
2. Stir until smooth, If too thick, thin with a bit of water.
3. Refrigerate in an airtight container for at least 5 days.

NUTRITION

Calories: 1059 Kcal; Protein: 27 g; Carbohydrates: 5 g; Fat: 90 g

TZATZIKI—CUCUMBER YOGURT SAUCE

8 minutes

0 minutes

2

INGREDIENTS

- ⅓ cup olive oil
- ⅔ cup Coconut Yogurt
- 2 cups cucumber, roughly chopped, seedless (1 large cucumber)
- 2 garlic cloves, peeled
- Juice of 2 lemons
- 1 tbsp dill weed, dried
- 1 tsp fine Himalayan salt
- 1½ tsp black pepper, ground

DIRECTIONS

1. In a blender, add all the ingredients and blend until smooth.
2. Place in a glass jar with a tight-fitting lid, and store in the refrigerator for up to 1 week. Shake well and use.

NUTRITION

Calories: 547 Kcal; Protein: 4 g; Carbohydrate: 8 g; Fat: 54 g

GARLICKY HONEY-MUSTARD SAUCE WITH SESAME OIL

INGREDIENTS

- ½ cup raw honey or maple syrup
- ½ cup Dijon mustard
- 1 tsp sesame oil, toasted
- 1 garlic clove, minced

DIRECTIONS

1. Add the honey, Dijon, sesame oil, and garlic to a small bowl, and whisk until combined.
2. Store in an airtight container and chill in the refrigerator.

NUTRITION

Calories: 420 Kcal; Protein: 1 g; Carbohydrates: 87 g; Fat: 1 g

10 minutes

0 minutes

1

HEALTHY AVOCADO DRESSING

INGREDIENTS

- ¼ cup yogurt
- ¼ tsp coriander
- 1 tbsp lemon juice
- 1 ripe avocado
- 1 green onion, chopped

DIRECTIONS

1. Put the avocado, yogurt, lemon juice, green onion, and coriander in a food processor and stir at high speed until smooth.
2. Put the mixture in an airtight container, close the lid, and put it in the refrigerator.

NUTRITION

Calories: 385 Kcal; Protein: 10 g; Carbohydrates: 27 g; Fat: 19 g

10 minutes

5 minutes

2 cups

SIMPLE BERRY VINAIGRETTE

15 minutes

5 minutes

1 ½ cups

INGREDIENTS

- ½ cup balsamic vinegar
- 1 tbsp lemon or lime zest
- 2 tbsp lemon or lime juice, freshly squeezed
- ⅓ cup extra-virgin olive oil
- 1 cup berries, fresh or frozen, no added sugar (thawed if frozen)
- 1 tbsp raw honey or maple syrup
- 1 tsp salt
- ½ tsp black pepper, freshly ground
- 1 tbsp Dijon mustard

DIRECTIONS

1. Put the berries, balsamic vinegar, olive oil, lemon juice, honey, lemon zest, Dijon mustard, salt, and pepper in a blender, and beat into a puree.
2. Put the puree in an airtight container and put it in the refrigerator for up to 5 days.

NUTRITION

Calories: 730 Kcal; Protein: 1 g; Carbohydrates: 19 g; Fat: 72 g

---

BARBECUE TAHINI SAUCE

5 minutes

0 minutes

8

INGREDIENTS

- 6 tbsp tahini sauce
- ¾ tsp garlic powder
- ⅛ tsp red chili powder
- 2 tsp maple syrup
- ¼ tsp salt
- 3 tsp molasses
- 3 tsp apple cider vinegar
- ¼ tsp liquid smoke
- 10 tsp tomato paste
- ½ cup of water

DIRECTIONS

1. Place all the ingredients in the order in a food processor or blender and then pulse for 3 to 5 minutes at high speed until smooth.
2. Pour the sauce into a bowl and then serve.

NUTRITION

Calories: 445 Kcal; Protein: 9 g; Carbohydrates: 85 g; Fat: 7 g

BOLOGNESE SAUCE

INGREDIENTS

- ½ small green bell pepper, chopped
- 1 stalk celery, chopped
- 1 small carrot, chopped
- 1 medium white onion, peeled, chopped
- 2 tsp garlic, minced
- ½ tsp red pepper flakes, crushed
- 3 tbsp olive oil
- 8-oz. tempeh, crumbled
- 8 oz. white mushrooms, chopped
- ½ cup red lentils, dried
- 28-oz. whole tomatoes, chopped
- 1 tsp oregano, dried
- ½ tsp fennel seed
- ½ tsp black pepper, ground
- ½ tsp salt
- 1 tsp basil, dried
- ¼ cup parsley, chopped
- 1 bay leaf
- 6-oz. tomato paste
- 1 cup dry red wine

DIRECTIONS

1. Take a Dutch oven, place it over medium heat, add oil, and when hot, add the first 6 ingredients, stir and cook: for 5 minutes until sauté.
2. Then switch heat to medium-high level, add the 2 ingredients after the olive oil, stir and cook for 3 minutes.
3. Switch heat to medium-low level, stir in tomato paste, and continue cooking for 2 minutes.
4. Add the remaining ingredients except for lentils, stir and bring the mixture to a boil.
5. Switch heat to the low level, simmer sauce for 10 minutes, covering the pan partially, then add lentils and continue cooking for 20 minutes until tender.
6. Serve sauce with cooked pasta.

55 minutes

0 minutes

8

NUTRITION

Calories: 978 Kcal; Protein: 72 g; Carbohydrates: 154 g; Fat: 27 g

---

CHIPOTLE BEAN CHEESY DIP

INGREDIENTS

- 2 cups pinto beans, cooked, mashed
- 1 tbsp chipotle chiles in adobo, minced
- ¼ cup of water
- ½ cup vegan cheddar cheese, shredded
- ¾ cup tomato salsa
- 1 tsp chili powder
- Salt

DIRECTIONS

1. In a bowl combine the mashed beans, chipotle chili, salsa, chili powder, and water in an instant pot.
2. Mix well and cover with a lid.
3. Cook for about 5 minutes.
4. Add the cheddar cheese and salt and serve warm.
5. Drain the tomatoes and add them to a blender.

10 minutes

0 minutes

3 cups

NUTRITION

Calories: 585 Kcal; Protein: 30 g; Carbohydrates: 90 g; Fat: 9 g

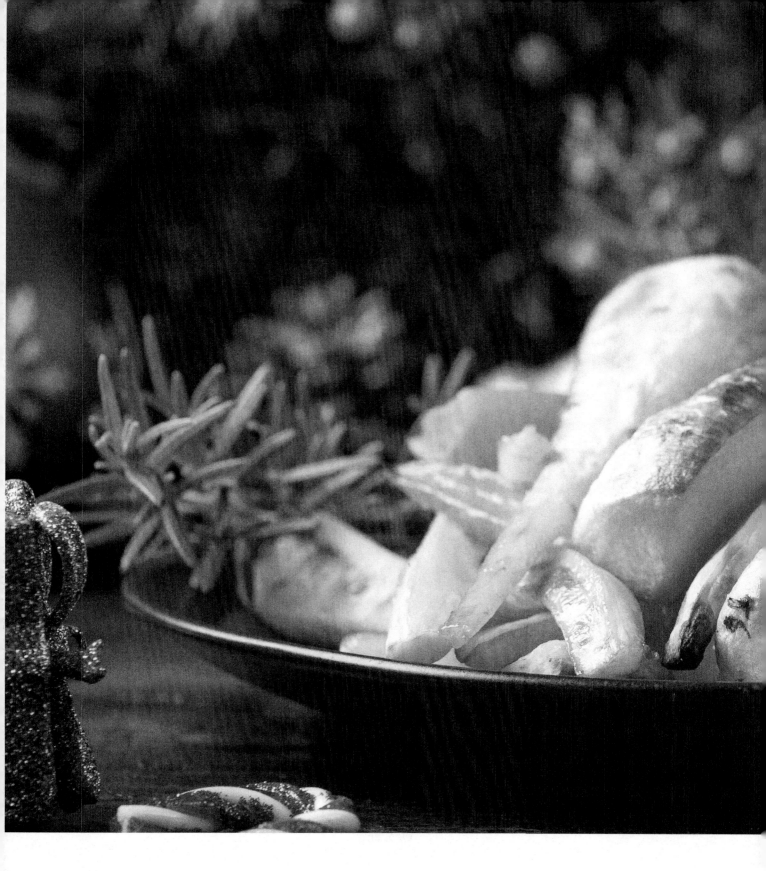

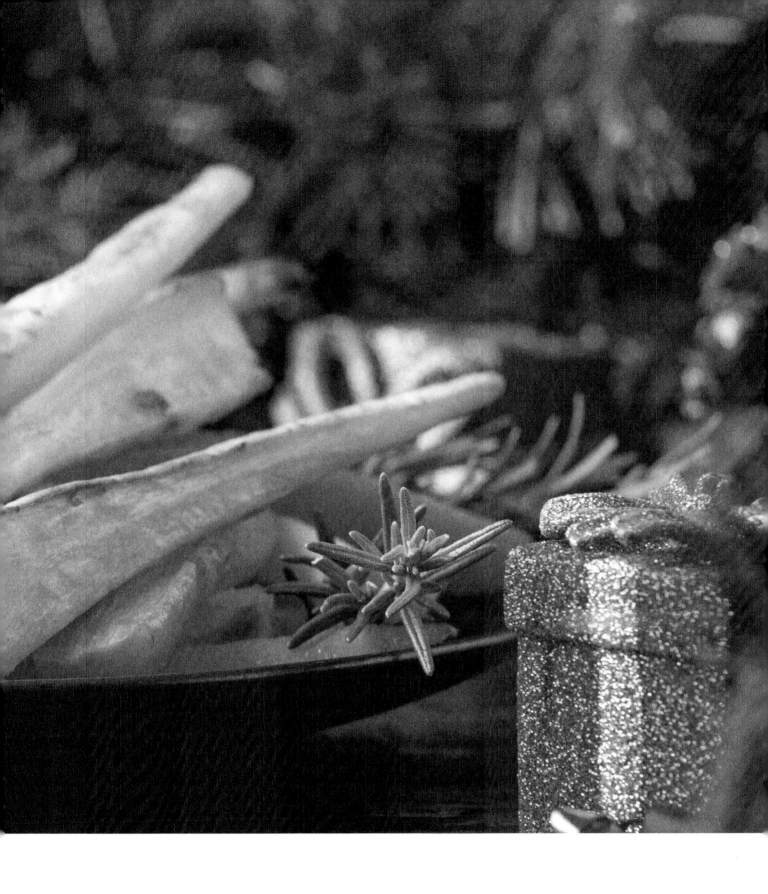

CHAPTER 10
SIDE DISHES

THYME WITH HONEY-ROASTED CARROTS

5 minutes

30 minutes

4

INGREDIENTS

- 1/5 lb. carrots, with the tops
- 1 tbsp honey
- 2 tbsp olive oil
- ½ tsp thyme, dried
- ½ tsp sea salt

DIRECTIONS

1. Preheat your oven to 425°F.
2. Lay parchment paper on your baking sheet.
3. Toss your carrots with honey, oil, thyme, and salt. Coat well.
4. Keep in a single layer. Bake in your oven for 30 minutes.
5. Set aside for cooling before serving.

NUTRITION

Calories: 209 Kcal; Protein: 1 g; Carbohydrates: 19 g; Fat: 9 g

---

ROASTED PARSNIPS

5 minutes

30 minutes

4

INGREDIENTS

- 1 tbsp extra-virgin olive oil
- 1 lb. parsnips
- 1 tsp kosher salt
- 1-½ tsp Italian seasoning
- Parsley, chopped, for garnishing

DIRECTIONS

1. Preheat your oven to 400°F.
2. Peel the parsnips. Cut them into 1" chunks.
3. Now toss with the seasoning, salt, and oil in a bowl.
4. Spread this on your baking sheet. It should be in one layer.
5. Roast for 30 minutes. Stir every 10 minutes.
6. Transfer to a plate. Garnish with parsley.

NUTRITION

Calories: 459 Kcal; Protein: 9 g; Carbohydrates: 43 g; Fat: 14 g

GREEN BEANS

INGREDIENTS

- ½ tsp red pepper flakes
- 2 tbsp extra-virgin olive oil
- 2 garlic cloves, minced
- 1-½ lb. green beans, trimmed
- 2 tbsp water
- ½ tsp kosher salt

DIRECTIONS

1. Heat oil in a skillet at medium temperature.
2. Include the pepper flake. Stir to coat in the olive oil.
3. Include the green beans. Cook for 7 minutes.
4. Stir often. The beans should be brown in some areas.
5. Add the salt and garlic. Cook for 1 minute, while stirring.
6. Pour water and cover immediately.
7. Cook covered for 1 more minute.

5 minutes

10 minutes

5

NUTRITION

Calories: 273 Kcal; Protein: 8 g; Carbohydrates: 32 g; Fat: 16 g

---

TEX-MEX COLE SLAW

INGREDIENTS

- 2 cups black beans, cooked
- 1.5 cups grape tomatoes, sliced in half
- 1.5 cups grilled corn kernels
- 1 jalapeno, seeded and minced
- 0.5 cup cilantro, chopped
- 1 bell pepper, diced
- 16 oz. coleslaw cabbage mix
- 3 tbsp lime juice
- 0.6 cup light sour cream
- 1 cup olive oil mayonnaise, reduced fat
- 1 tbsp chili powder
- 1 tsp cumin, ground
- 1 tsp onion powder
- 1 tsp garlic powder

DIRECTIONS

1. Mix the sour cream, mayonnaise, lime juice, garlic powder, onion powder, cumin, and chili powder in a bowl to create the dressing.
2. In a large bowl, toss the vegetables and then add in the prepared dressing and toss again until evenly coated. Chill the mixture in the fridge for 30 minutes to 12 hours before serving.

15 minutes

0 minutes

12

NUTRITION

Calories: 1348 Kcal; Protein: 48 g; Carbohydrates: 143 g; Fat: 54 g

ROASTED OKRA

15 minutes

20 minutes

4

INGREDIENTS

- 1 lb. okra, fresh
- 2 tbsp extra virgin olive oil
- 5 tsp cayenne pepper, ground
- 1 tsp paprika
- 0.25 tsp garlic powder

DIRECTIONS

1. Warm the oven to 450°F and prepare a large baking sheet. Cut the okra into pieces appropriate ½" in size.
2. Place the okra on the baking pan and top it with olive oil and seasonings, giving it a good toss until evenly coated. Roast the okra in the heated oven until it is tender and lightly browned and seared. Serve immediately while hot.

NUTRITION

Calories: 150 Kcal; Protein: 9 g; Carbohydrates: 33 g; Fat: 5 g

BROWN SUGAR GLAZED CARROTS

15 minutes

25 minutes

6

INGREDIENTS

- 2 lb. carrots, sliced into 1" pieces
- 0.3 cup light olive oil
- 0.5 cup Truvia brown sugar blend
- 1 tsp black pepper, ground

DIRECTIONS

1. Warm the oven to 400°F and prepare a large baking sheet. Toss the carrots with the oil, Truvia, and black pepper until evenly coated, and then spread them out on the prepared baking sheet.
2. Place the carrots in the oven and allow them to roast until tender, about 20 to 25 minutes. Halfway through the cooking time, turn them over.. Remove the carrots from the oven and serve them alone or topped with fresh parsley.

NUTRITION

Calories: 377 Kcal; Protein: 8 g; Carbohydrates: 89 g; Fat: 3 g

OVEN-ROASTED BEETS WITH HONEY RICOTTA

INGREDIENTS

- 1 lb. purple beets
- 1 lb. golden beets
- 0.5 cup ricotta cheese, low-fat
- 3 tbsp extra virgin olive oil
- 1 tbsp honey
- 1 tsp rosemary, fresh, chopped
- 0.5 tsp black pepper, ground

DIRECTIONS

1. Warm the oven to 375°F and prepare a large baking sheet by lining it with kitchen parchment. Slice the beets into ½" cubes before tossing them with the extra virgin olive oil and black pepper.
2. Put the beets on the prepared baking sheet and allow them to roast until tender, about 35 to 40 minutes. Halfway through the cooking process, flip the beets over.
3. Meanwhile, in a small bowl, whisk the ricotta with the rosemary and honey. Refrigerate until ready to serve. Once the beets are done cooking, serve them topped with the ricotta mixture, and enjoy.

15 minutes

40 minutes

6

NUTRITION

Calories: 470 Kcal; Protein: 21 g; Carbohydrates: 88 g; Fat: 8 g

EASY CARROTS MIX

INGREDIENTS

- 15 carrots, halved lengthwise
- 2 tbsp coconut sugar
- ¼ cup olive oil
- ½ tsp rosemary, dried
- ½ tsp garlic powder
- A pinch of black pepper

DIRECTIONS

1. In a bowl, combine the carrots with the sugar, oil, rosemary, garlic powder, and black pepper, toss well, spread on a lined baking sheet, and place in the oven and bake at 400°F for 40 minutes.
2. Serve.

10 minutes

40 minutes

6

NUTRITION

Calories: 486 Kcal; Protein: 11 g; Carbohydrates: 112 g; Fat: 3 g

124

10 minutes

6 minutes

4

TASTY GRILLED ASPARAGUS

INGREDIENTS

- 2 lb. asparagus, trimmed
- 2 tbsp olive oil
- A pinch of salt and black pepper

DIRECTIONS

1. In a bowl, combine the asparagus with salt, pepper, and oil and toss well.
2. Place the asparagus on a preheated grill over medium-high heat, cook for 3 minutes on each side, then serve.

NUTRITION

Calories: 181 Kcal; Protein: 21 g; Carbohydrates: 35 g; Fat: 1 g

125

10 minutes

5 hours

10

LIMA BEANS DISH

INGREDIENTS

- 1 green bell pepper, chopped
- 1 sweet red pepper, chopped
- 1 and ½ cups tomato sauce, salt-free
- 1 yellow onion, chopped
- ½ cup of water
- 16 oz. kidney beans, canned, no-salt-added, drained, and rinsed
- 16 oz. black-eyed peas, canned, no-salt-added, drained, and rinsed
- 15 oz. corn
- 15 oz. lima beans, canned, no-salt-added, drained, and rinsed
- 15 oz. black beans, canned, no-salt-added, and drained
- 2 celery ribs, chopped
- 2 bay leaves
- 1 tsp mustard, ground
- 1 tbsp cider vinegar

DIRECTIONS

1. In a slow cooker, mix the tomato sauce with the celery, onion, green bell pepper, water, red pepper bay leaves, vinegar, mustard, kidney beans, corn, black-eyed peas, lima beans, and black beans, cook on Low for 5 hours.
2. Discard bay leaves, divide the whole mix between plates, and serve.

NUTRITION

Calories: 1320 Kcal; Protein: 72 g; Carbohydrates: 246 g; Fat: 13 g

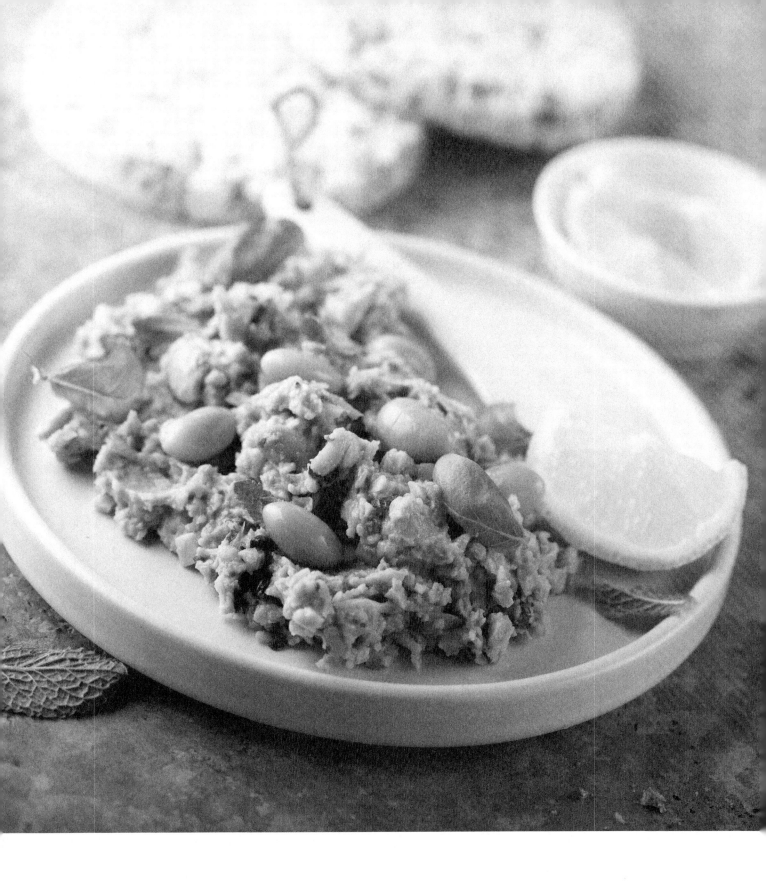

BaKED JICaMa FRIES

20 minutes

50 minutes

4

INGREDIENTS

- 1-lb. jicama root
- 2 tbsp butter
- 1 tbsp extra-virgin olive oil
- 1 tsp chili powder
- 1 tsp paprika
- ¼ tsp salt
- ⅛ tsp black pepper, freshly ground
- 2 tbsp Parmesan cheese, grated

DIRECTIONS

1. Peel the jicama and cut into ½" slices. Cut the slices into strips, each about 4"long.
2. In a large saucepan, place the jicama strips and cover them with water. Bring to a boil, then boil for 9 minutes. Drain the jicama well and transfer to a rimmed baking sheet. Pat the strips with a paper towel while waiting for them to be dry so that the strips will crisp in the oven.
3. Preheat the oven to 400°F.
4. In a mini saucepan, melt the butter with olive oil. Drizzle over the jicama on the baking sheet. Sprinkle with the chili powder, paprika, salt, and pepper, and toss to coat. Spread the strips into a single layer.
5. Bake the jicama fries for 40 to 45 minutes or until they are browned and crisp, turning once with a spatula halfway through the cooking time.
6. Sprinkle with the Parmesan cheese and serve.

NUTRITION

Calories: 249 Kcal; Protein: 5 g; Carbohydrates: 40 g; Fat: 8 g

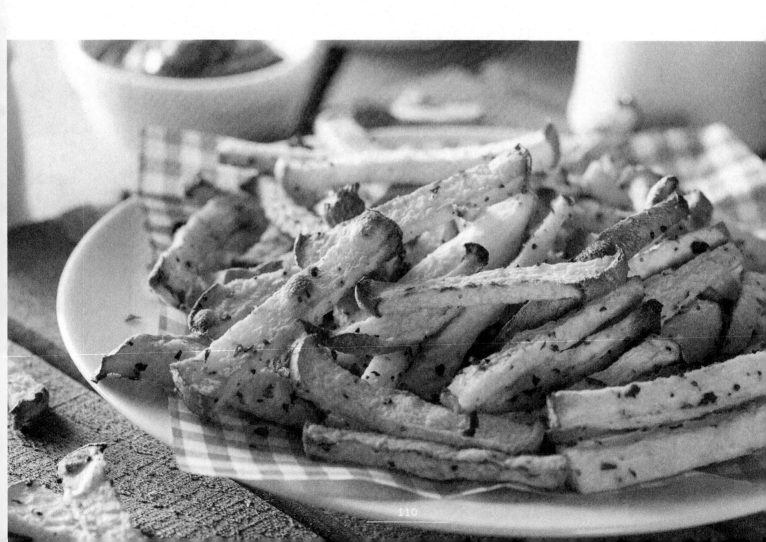

DOUBLE-BOILED SWEET POTATOES

INGREDIENTS

- 2 large, sweet potatoes, peeled and cut into 1-" cubes
- 2 tbsp extra-virgin olive oil
- 2 tbsp butter
- 1 red onion, chopped
- 1 tbsp honey
- ¼ tsp salt
- ⅛ tsp black pepper, freshly ground

DIRECTIONS

1. In a large saucepan, fill the pot with water to about an inch above the potatoes. Add the sweet potato cubes and bring to a boil. Boil for 10 minutes.
2. Drain the sweet potatoes, discarding the water.
3. In the same saucepan, fill the pot to the same level again. Add the sweet potato cubes and bring to a boil for 10 to 15 minutes, or until the potatoes are tender.
4. In the meantime, in a large frying pan, heat the olive oil and butter. Add the red onion and cook for 3 to 5 minutes, stirring, until the onion is very tender.
5. Drain the sweet potatoes once more, discarding the water again. Add the sweet potatoes to your skillet along with the half-and-half, honey, salt, and pepper.
6. Pound the potatoes, using an immersion blender or a potato masher, until the desired consistency. Serve.

NUTRITION

Calories: 545 Kcal; Protein: 5 g; Carbohydrates: 66 g; Fat: 25 g

20 minutes

25 minutes

4

EDAMAME GUACAMOLE

INGREDIENTS

- 1 cup edamame, thawed, frozen, shelled
- ¼ cup of water
- Juice and zest of 1 lemon
- 2 tbsp fresh cilantro, chopped
- 1 tbsp olive oil
- 1 tsp garlic, minced

DIRECTIONS

1. In your food processor or blender, blend the edamame, water, lemon juice, lemon zest, cilantro, olive oil, and garlic, and pulse until blended but still a bit chunky.
2. Serve fresh.

NUTRITION

Calories: 167 Kcal; Protein: 9 g; Carbohydrates: 21 g; Fat: 5 g

10 minutes

0 minutes

4

129

15 minutes

3 to 4 hours

4

TOASTED PEAR CHIPS

INGREDIENTS

- Olive oil cooking spray
- 4 firm pears, cored and cut into ⅛"-thick slices
- 2 tsp cinnamon, ground
- 1 tbsp sugar

DIRECTIONS

1. Preheat the oven to 200°F.
2. Line a baking sheet with parchment paper, then lightly coat with cooking spray.
3. Spread the pear slices on the baking sheet with no overlap.
4. Sprinkle with the cinnamon and sugar.
5. Bake until the chips are dry, 3 to 4 hours. Cool completely.
6. Store in a sealed container for up to 4 days in a cool, dark place.

NUTRITION

Calories: 264 Kcal; Protein: 2 g; Carbohydrates: 57 g; Fat: 0 g

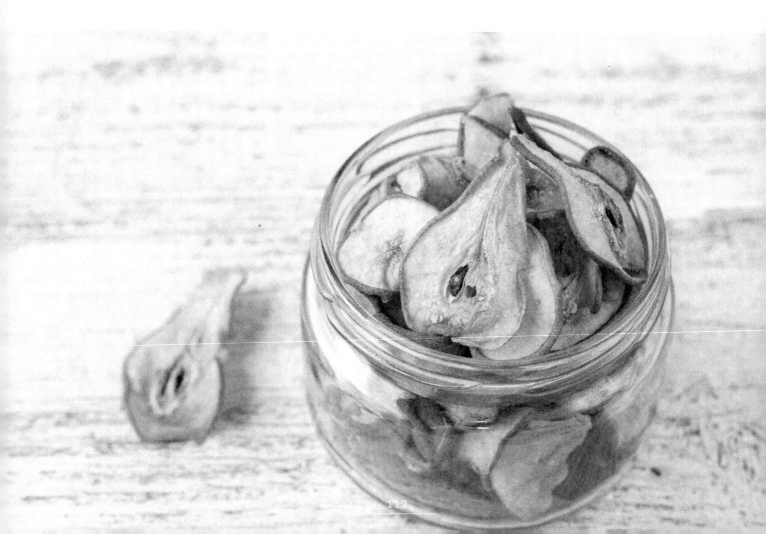

CITRUS SESAME COOKIES

INGREDIENTS

- ¾ cup unsalted butter, at room temperature
- ½ cup sugar
- 1 egg
- 1 tsp vanilla extract
- 2 cups all-purpose flour
- 2 tbsp sesame seeds, toasted
- ½ tsp baking soda
- 1 tsp lemon zest, freshly grated
- 1 tsp orange zest, freshly grated

DIRECTIONS

1. Pulse together the margarine and sugar on high speed until thick and fluffy, around 3 minutes.
2. Add the egg and vanilla, then beat to mix carefully, grinding down the sides of the bowl.
3. In a small container, stir together the flour, sesame seeds, baking soda, lemon zest, and orange zest.
4. Put the flour mix into the butter mixture and stir until well blended.
5. Roll the dough into a long cylinder around 2"in diameter and wrap it in plastic wrap. Chill for an hour.
6. Turn on the oven to 350°F.
7. Line a baking sheet with parchment paper.
8. Cut the firm cookie dough into ½"-thick rounds and place them on the prepared baking sheet.
9. Bake for around 10 to 12 minutes until lightly golden. Cool completely on wire racks.
10. Place in a sealed container and store in the refrigerator for up to 1 week. You can also store it in the freezer for up to 2 months.

15 minutes

10 minutes

18

NUTRITION

Calories: 2152 Kcal; Protein: 176 g; Carbohydrates: 16 g; Fat: 141 g

CRUNCHY CHICKEN SALAD WRAPS

INGREDIENTS

- 8 oz. chicken, cooked and shredded
- 1 scallion, white and green parts, chopped
- ½ cup red grapes, halved and seedless
- 1 celery stalk, chopped
- ¼ cup low-sodium mayonnaise or store-bought mayonnaise
- Pinch black pepper, freshly ground
- 4 large lettuce leaves, butter or red leaf

DIRECTIONS

1. In your medium-sized bowl, stir together the chicken, scallion, grapes, celery, and mayonnaise until mixed.
2. Season the mixture with pepper.
3. Spoon the chicken salad onto the lettuce leaves and serve.

15 minutes

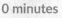

0 minutes

4

NUTRITION

Calories: 346 Kcal; Protein: 43 g; Carbohydrates: 6 g; Fat: 13 g

WILD MUSHROOM COUSCOUS

15 minutes

10 minutes

5

INGREDIENTS

- 1 tbsp olive oil
- 1 cup mixed wild mushrooms (shiitake, cremini, Portobello, oyster, enoki)
- ¼ sweet onion, finely chopped
- 1 tsp garlic, minced
- 1 tbsp fresh oregano, chopped
- 3½ cups of water
- 10 oz. couscous

DIRECTIONS

1. Put the olive oil in a large fry pan over medium-high heat.
2. Add the mushrooms, onion, and garlic, and sauté until tender, about 6 minutes.
3. Stir in the oregano and water and bring the mixture to a boil.
4. Remove the saucepan from the heat and stir in the couscous.
5. Cover the pan and allow it to stand for 5 minutes.
6. Fluff the couscous with a fork and serve.

NUTRITION

Calories: 269 Kcal; Protein: 12 g; Carbohydrates: 44 g; Fat: 3 g

---

SAUTÉED BUTTERNUT SQUASH

10 minutes

20 minutes

8

INGREDIENTS

- 1 tbsp olive oil
- 4 cups 1" cubes butternut squash, peeled, seeded
- ½ sweet onion, chopped
- 1 tsp fresh thyme, chopped
- Pinch black pepper, freshly ground

DIRECTIONS

1. Put the olive oil in a large frying pan over medium-high heat..
2. Add the butternut squash and sauté until tender, about 15 minutes.
3. Add the onion and thyme, and sauté for 5 minutes.
4. Season with pepper and serve hot.

NUTRITION

Calories: 373 Kcal; Protein: 8 g; Carbohydrates: 90 g; Fat: 7 g

HERB ROASTED CAULIFLOWER

INGREDIENTS

- 1 tbsp olive oil, plus more for the pan
- 1 head cauliflower, cut in half and then into ½"-thick slices
- 1 tsp fresh thyme, chopped
- 1 tsp fresh chives, chopped
- ¼ tsp black pepper, freshly ground

DIRECTIONS

1. Preheat the oven to 400°F.
2. Lightly coat a baking sheet with olive oil.
3. Toss the cauliflower, 1 tbsp of olive oil, the thyme, chives, and pepper until well coated.
4. Spread the cauliflower on the prepared baking sheet.
5. Roast, turning once, until both sides are golden, for about 20 minutes.

NUTRITION

Calories: 244 Kcal; Protein: 10 g; Carbohydrates: 40 g; Fat: 7 g

10 minutes

20 minutes

4

TASTY CHICKEN MEATBALLS

INGREDIENTS

- ½ lb. chicken, lean ground
- ¼ cup breadcrumbs
- 1 scallion, white and green parts, chopped
- 1 egg, beaten
- 1 tsp garlic, minced
- ¼ tsp black pepper, freshly ground
- Pinch red pepper flakes

DIRECTIONS

1. Preheat the oven to 400°F.
2. In a large bowl, blend the chicken, breadcrumbs, scallion, egg, garlic, black pepper, and red pepper flakes.
3. Form the chicken mixture into 18 meatballs and place them on a baking sheet.
4. Bake the meatballs for about 25 minutes, turning several times, until golden brown.
5. Serve hot.

NUTRITION

Calories: 386 Kcal; Protein: 48 g; Carbohydrates: 3 g; Fat: 30 g

10 minutes

25 minutes

6

136

10 minutes + 4 hours

0 minute

MARINATED FETA AND ARTICHOKES

3

INGREDIENTS

- 4 oz. traditional Greek feta, cut into ½" cubes
- 4 oz. artichoke hearts, drained, quartered lengthwise
- ⅓ cup extra-virgin olive oil
- Zest and juice of 1 lemon
- 2 tbsp fresh rosemary, roughly chopped
- 2 tbsp fresh parsley, roughly chopped
- ½ tsp black peppercorns

DIRECTIONS

1. In a glass bowl, combine the feta and artichoke hearts. Add the olive oil, lemon zest and juice, rosemary, parsley, and peppercorns, and toss gently to coat, being sure not to crumble the feta.
2. Cover and chill for 4 hours before serving.

NUTRITION

Calories:347 Kcal; Protein: 4 g; Carbohydrates: 11 g; Fat: 23 g

---

137

10' + 4h

0 minute

4

CITRUS-MARINATED OLIVES

INGREDIENTS

- 2 cups mixed green olives with pits
- ¼ cup red wine vinegar
- ¼ cup extra-virgin olive oil
- 2 garlic cloves, finely minced
- Zest and juice orange
- 1 tsp red pepper flakes
- 2 bay leaves
- ½ tsp cumin, ground
- ½ tsp allspice, ground

DIRECTIONS

1. In a jar, mix olives, vinegar, oil, garlic, orange zest and juice, red pepper flakes, bay leaves, cumin, and allspice.
2. Cover and chill for 4 hours, tossing again before serving.

NUTRITION

Calories:167 Kcal; Protein: 3 g; Carbohydrates: 12 g; Fat: 16 g

BALSAMIC ARTICHOKE ANTIPASTO

INGREDIENTS

- 1 (12-oz./340-g) jar of red peppers, roasted, steamed, drained and seeded
- 1 (16-oz./454-g) can of garbanzo beans, drained
- 8 artichoke hearts, either jarred, drained, or frozen (thawed)
- 1 cup whole Kalamata olives, drained
- ¼ cup balsamic vinegar
- ½ tsp salt

DIRECTIONS

1. Slice the peppers into ½" slices and place them into a large bowl.
2. Slice the artichoke hearts into quarters and add them to the bowl.
3. Add the olives, garbanzo beans, salt, and balsamic vinegar.
4. Toss all the ingredients together. Serve chilled.

NUTRITION

Calories: 1127 Kcal; Protein: 21 g; Carbohydrates: 110 g; Fat: 50 g

5 minutes

0 minutes

4

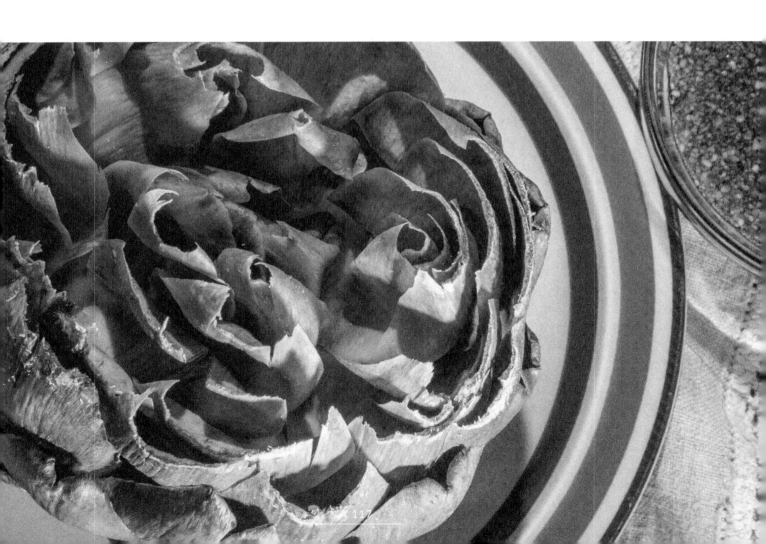

139

MASCARPONE PECANS STUFFED DATES

5 minutes

5 minutes

12 to 15

INGREDIENTS

- 1 cup pecans, shells removed
- 1 (8-oz.) container of Mascarpone cheese
- 20 Medjool dates

DIRECTIONS

1. Let the oven heat to 350°F (180°C). Place the pecans on a baking sheet and bake for about 5 to 6 minutes, until aromatic and lightly toasted. Get the pecans out of the oven and cool them for 5 minutes.
2. Once chilled, place the pecans in a food processor fitted with a chopping blade and chop until they bear a resemblance to the texture of coarse sugar or bulgur wheat.
3. Reserve ¼ cup of ground pecans in a mini bowl. Pour the remaining chopped pecans into a bigger bowl and add the Mascarpone cheese.
4. Mix the cheese with the pecans until evenly combined using a spatula.
5. Ladle the cheese mixture into a piping bag.
6. Cut one side of the date lengthwise, from the stem to the bottom using a knife. Slightly open and remove the pit.
7. Squeeze a substantial amount of the cheese mixture into the date where the pit used to be using the piping bag. Close up the date and repeat with the rest of the dates.
8. Dip any visible cheese from the stuffed dates into the reserved chopped pecans to cover it up.
9. Put the dates on a serving plate; serve immediately or chill in the fridge until you are ready to serve.

NUTRITION

Calories: 2533 Kcal; Protein: 28 g; Carbohydrates: 361 g; Fat: 121 g

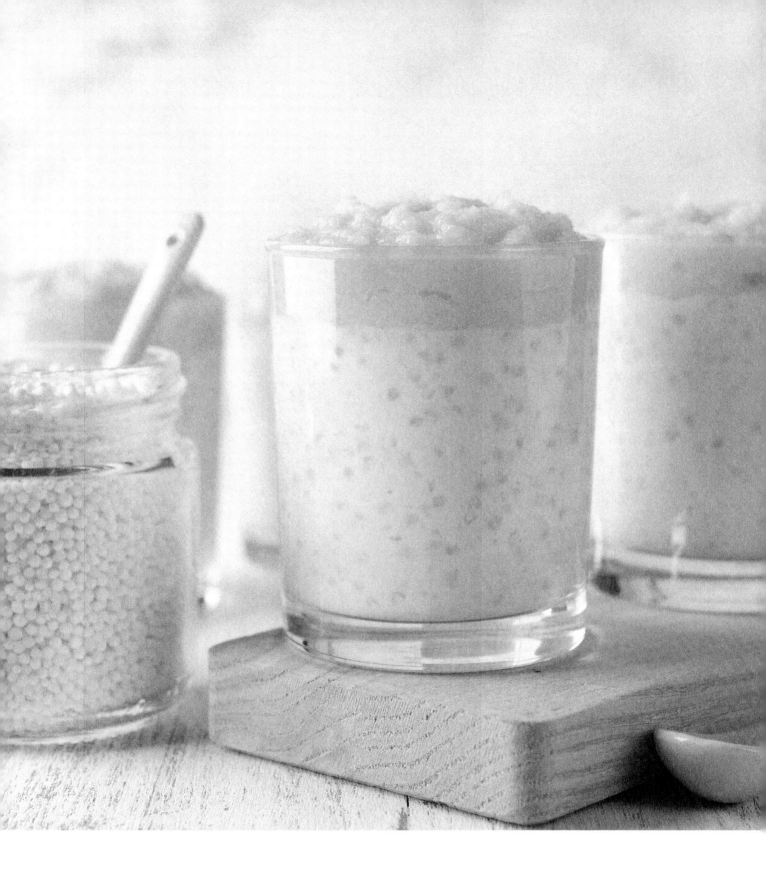

HEALTHY BROCCOLI MUFFINS

5 minutes

30 minutes

6

INGREDIENTS

- 12 eggs, whisked
- 1 tbsp Coconut oil
- 1 cup broccoli, chopped
- 1 small onion, chopped
- Pepper
- Sea salt

DIRECTIONS

1. Grease muffin tray with coconut oil.
2. Divide evenly broccoli and onion in the muffin tray.
3. Now divide evenly eggs in the muffin tray.
4. Season with pepper and salt.
5. Bake at 400°F/204°C for 15 minutes.

NUTRITION

Calories: 925 Kcal; Protein: 77 g; Carbohydrates: 10 g; Fat:61 g

---

SIMPLE ZUCCHINI MUFFINS

5 minutes

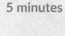

40 minutes

5

INGREDIENTS

- Coconut oil as needed
- 1 cup zucchini, shredded
- 3 eggs
- 1 cup almond flour
- ¼ tsp sea salt

DIRECTIONS

1. Grease muffin tray with coconut oil.
2. Add all ingredients to your blender, and blend until mixed.
3. Pour into grease muffin tray and bake at 350°F/176°C for 25 minutes.
4. Serve warm and enjoy.

NUTRITION

Calories: 913 Kcal; Protein: 45 g; Carbohydrates: 27 g; Fat: 75 g

FIG AND HONEY BUCKWHEAT PUDDING

INGREDIENTS

- ½ tsp cinnamon, ground
- ½ cup figs, dried and chopped
- ⅓ cup honey
- 1 tsp pure vanilla extract
- 3 ½ cups milk
- ½ tsp pure almond extract
- 1 ½ cups buckwheat

DIRECTIONS

1. Add all the above ingredients to your Instant Pot.
2. Secure the lid. Choose the "Multigrain" mode and cook for 10 minutes under high pressure. Once cooking is complete, use a natural pressure release; carefully remove the lid.
3. Serve topped with fresh fruits, nuts, or whipped topping. Bon appétit!

NUTRITION

Calories: 320 Kcal; Protein: 9 g; Carbohydrates: 57 g; Fat: 7 g

10 minutes

10 minutes

4

ZINGY BLUEBERRY SAUCE

INGREDIENTS

- ¼ cup fresh lemon juice
- ½ -lb. sugar, granulated
- 1 tbsp lemon zest, freshly grated
- ½ tsp vanilla extract
- 1 lb. fresh blueberries

DIRECTIONS

1. Place the blueberries, sugar, and vanilla in the inner pot of your Instant Pot.
2. Secure the lid. Choose the "Manual" mode and cook for 2 minutes at high pressure. Once cooking is complete, use a natural pressure release for 15 minutes; carefully remove the lid.
3. Stir in the lemon zest and juice. Puree in a food processor; then, strain and push the mixture through a sieve before storing. Enjoy!

NUTRITION

Calories: 1166 Kcal; Protein: 3 g; Carbohydrates: 293 g; Fat: 3 g

5 minutes

20 minutes

10

SMALL PUMPKIN PASTRY CREAM

5 minutes

10 minutes

8

INGREDIENTS

- 1 can (16 oz.) pumpkin, prepared
- 1 (14-oz.) can of milk, sweetened and condensed
- 3 eggs, beaten
- 1 tsp polished ginger, finely chopped (optional)
- 1 tsp cinnamon, ground
- ¼ tsp cloves, ground
- 1 cup of water

DIRECTIONS

1. Mix the pumpkin, milk, eggs, cinnamon, ginger, and cloves. Pour into individual cups for custard.
2. Cover each cup firmly with the foil. Pour the water into the pot. Position the cups on the rack of the pot. Close and secure the lid.
3. Put the pressure regulator on the vent tube and cook for 10 minutes once the pressure regulator begins to rock slowly. Cool the pot quickly. Let the cream cool well in the refrigerator. If desired, serve with whipped cream.

NUTRITION

Calories: 476 Kcal; Protein: 3 0 g; Carbohydrates: 43 g; Fat: 21 g

---

TAPIOCA PUDDING

5 minutes

20 minutes

6

INGREDIENTS

- 2 cups of low-fat milk
- 2 tbsp quick-cooking tapioca
- 2 eggs, lightly beaten
- ⅓ cup sugar
- ½ tsp vanilla
- 1 cup of water

DIRECTIONS

1. Heat the milk and tapioca. Remove from heat then let stand for 15 minutes.
2. Combine eggs, sugar, and vanilla. Add milk and tapioca, stirring constantly.
3. Pour them into individual cups for custard. Cover each cup firmly with the foil. Pour the water into the pot.
4. Position the cups on the rack of the pot. Close and secure the lid.
5. Place the pressure regulator on the vent tube and cook for 5 minutes once the pressure regulator begins to rock slowly.
6. Cool the pot quickly. Let the pudding cool well in the refrigerator.

NUTRITION

Calories: 375 Kcal; Protein: 30 g; Carbohydrates: 21 g; Fat: 18 g

GREEK-STYLE COMPOTE WITH YOGURT

INGREDIENTS

- 1 cup Greek yogurt
- 1 cup of pears
- 4 tbsp honey
- 1 cup of apples
- 1 vanilla bean
- 1 cinnamon stick
- ½ cup caster sugar
- 1 cup rhubarb
- 1 tsp ginger, ground
- 1 cup of plums

DIRECTIONS

1. Place the fruits, ginger, vanilla, cinnamon, and caster sugar in the inner pot of your Instant Pot.
2. Secure the lid. Choose the "Manual" mode and cook for 2 minutes at high pressure. Once cooking is complete, use a natural pressure release for 10 minutes; carefully remove the lid.
3. Meanwhile, whisk the yogurt with the honey.
4. Serve your compote in individual bowls with a dollop of honeyed Greek yogurt. Enjoy!

NUTRITION

Calories: 417 Kcal; Protein: 12 g; Carbohydrates: 92 g; Fat: 0 g

5 minutes

15 minutes

4

BUTTERSCOTCH LAVA CAKES

INGREDIENTS

- 7 tbsp all-purpose flour
- A pinch of coarse salt
- 6 oz. butterscotch morsels
- ¾ cup sugar, powdered
- ½ tsp vanilla extract
- 3 eggs, whisked
- 1 stick of butter
- 1 ½ cups of water

DIRECTIONS

1. Add 1 ½ cups water and a metal rack to the Instant Pot. Line a standard-size muffin tin with muffin papers.
2. In a microwave-safe bowl, microwave butter and butterscotch morsels for about 40 seconds. Stir in the powdered sugar.
3. Add the remaining ingredients. Spoon the batter into the prepared muffin tin.
4. Secure the lid. Choose the "Manual" and cook at High pressure for 10 minutes. Once cooking is complete, use a quick release; carefully remove the lid.
5. To remove, let it cool for 5–6 minutes. Run a small knife around the sides of each cake and serve. Enjoy!

5 minutes

15 minutes

6

NUTRITION

Calories: 393 Kcal; Protein: 5 g; Carbohydrates: 45 g; Fat: 21 g

VANILLA BREAD PUDDING WITH APRICOTS

5 minutes

15 minutes

6

INGREDIENTS

- 2 tbsp coconut oil
- ⅓ cup heavy cream
- 4 eggs, whisked
- ½ cup apricots, dried, soaked, and chopped
- 1 tsp cinnamon, ground
- ½ tsp star anise, ground
- A pinch of nutmeg, grated
- A pinch of salt
- ½ cup sugar, granulated
- 2 tbsp molasses
- 2 cups of milk
- 4 cups Italian bread, cubed
- 1 tsp vanilla paste
- 1 ½ cups of water

DIRECTIONS

1. Add 1 ½ cups water and a metal rack to the Instant Pot.
2. Grease a baking dish with a nonstick cooking spray. Throw the bread cubes into the prepared baking dish.
3. In a mixing bowl, thoroughly combine the remaining ingredients. Pour the mixture over the bread cubes. Cover with a piece of foil, making a foil sling.
4. Secure the lid. Choose the "Porridge" mode and high pressure; cook for 15 minutes. Once cooking is complete, use a quick pressure release; carefully remove the lid. Enjoy!

NUTRITION

Calories: 1082 Kcal; Protein: 43 g; Carbohydrates: 141 g; Fat: 38 g

---

MEDITERRANEAN-STYLE CARROT PUDDING

15 minutes

15 minutes

4

INGREDIENTS

- ⅓ cup almonds, ground
- ¼ cup figs, dried and chopped
- 2 large-sized carrots, shredded
- ½ cup of water
- ½ cup milk
- ½ tsp star anise, ground
- ⅓ tsp cardamom, ground
- ¼ tsp kosher salt
- ⅓ cup sugar, granulated
- 2 eggs, beaten
- ½ tsp pure almond extract
- ½ tsp vanilla extract
- ½ cup jasmine rice

DIRECTIONS

1. Place the jasmine rice, milk, water, carrots, and salt in your Instant Pot.
2. Stir to combine and secure the lid. Choose "Manual" and cook at high pressure for 10 minutes. Once cooking is complete, use a natural release for 15 minutes; carefully remove the lid.
3. Now, press the "Sauté" button and add the sugar, eggs, and almonds; stir to combine well. Bring to a boil; press the "Keep Warm/ Cancel" button.
4. Add the remaining ingredients and stir; the pudding will thicken as it sits. Bon appétit!

NUTRITION

Calories: 706 Kcal; Protein: 30 g; Carbohydrates: 75 g; Fat: 34 g

DAY	BREAKFAST	LUNCH	DINNER
1	Egg and Veggie Fajitas	Pan-Seared Haddock with Beets	Pesto Pork Chops
2	Fast Cabbage Cakes	Avocado-Orange Grilled Chicken	Fish Taco Salad with Strawberry Avocado Salsa
3	Green Vanilla Smoothie	Grilled Steak with Salsa	Avocado-Orange Grilled Chicken
4	Citrus Sesame Cookies	Spinach Sea Bass Lunch	Herbs and Lemony Roasted Chicken
5	Vanilla Turmeric Orange Juice	Lemon Chicken Mix	Baked Eggplant Slices
6	Peach Maple Smoothie	Vegan Chili	Beet Haddock Dinner
7	Healthy Broccoli Muffins	Oregano Pork	Hot Cabbage Quartet Salad
8	Honey Stewed Apples	Buckwheat Salad	Rosemary Pork Chops
9	Pistachio and Fruits	Fennel Baked Cod	Herbed Chicken
10	Simple Zucchini Muffins	Minty Olives and Tomatoes Salad	Brown Rice and Chicken Soup
11	Spicy Veggie Pancakes	Cod Cucumber Delight	Rosemary Pork Chops
12	Double-Boiled Sweet Potatoes	Cilantro Beef Curry with Cauliflower	Honey Scallops

13	Cucumber Kiwi Green Smoothie	Mexican Pepper Salmon	Beef Steaks with Creamy Bacon and Mushrooms
14	Crunchy Chicken Salad Wraps	Ground Chicken and Peas Curry	Spinach With Chickpeas and Lemon
15	Green Vanilla Smoothie	Herbs and Lemony Roasted Chicken	Pan-Seared Haddock with Beets
16	Pistachio and Fruits	Beans and Cucumber Salad	Oregano Pork
17	Citrus Sesame Cookies	Baked Eggplant Slices	Avocado-Orange Grilled Chicken
18	Cucumber Kiwi Green Smoothie	Buckwheat Salad	Vegan Chili
19	Crunchy Chicken Salad Wraps	Cilantro Beef Curry with Cauliflower	Hot Cabbage Quartet Salad
20	Double-Boiled Sweet Potatoes	Rosemary Pork Chops	Beet Haddock Dinner
21	Spicy Veggie Pancakes	Beef Steaks with Creamy Bacon and Mushrooms	Pesto Pork Chops

DISCOVER THE AMAZING BONUS I HAVE IN STORE FOR YOU

Scan the QR Code or go to www.vitaminsmineralsguides.com
for instant access to the 2 FREE life-saving guides that come with this Book:

FREE: A PRACTICAL 70+ PAGE GUIDEBOOK

Discover the vitamins and minerals that should never be missing from your diet – and which foods you can get them from –.

A free ultra-detailed report – suitable for beginners too – to discover all the essential nutrients for living a long and healthy life Here is everything you will find in this guide

» What are vitamins and why are they essential

» Minerals - what they do and why you should never be missing them in your diet-

» The 8 signs that you are deficient in vitamins or minerals and how to remedy that

» 3 facts that (maybe) you won't know about vitamins and minerals

» And much much more...

Printed in Great Britain
by Amazon